ELEGANCE

ELEGANCE

*Sleek, Chic and
At Their Peak:
Women After 40*

HELEN BULLOCK

Photographs by Jillian Edelstein

Hodder & Stoughton
LONDON SYDNEY AUCKLAND

*To Alexandra and Helen Mary Rose,
my elegant daughters, on their way
to becoming elegant women*

British Library Cataloguing in Publication Data

ISBN 0-340-56903-4

Copyright © Helen Bullock, 1992

Concept created by R. di R. Media Communications Ltd, 1992

First published in Great Britain 1992

All rights reserved. No part of this publication may be reproduced or transmitted in any form or by any means, electronic or mechanical, including photocopying, recording, or any information storage and retrieval system, without either prior permission in writing from the publisher or a licence permitting restricted copying. In the United Kingdom such licences are issued by the Copyright Licensing Agency, 90 Tottenham Court Road, London W1P 9HE. The right of Helen Bullock to be identified as the author of this work has been asserted by her in accordance with the Copyright, Designs and Patents Act 1988.

Published by Hodder and Stoughton,
a division of Hodder and Stoughton Ltd,
Mill Road, Dunton Green, Sevenoaks, Kent TN13 2YA
Editorial Office: 47 Bedford Square, London WC1B 3DB

Designed by Tim Higgins

Photoset by Rowland Phototypesetting Ltd,
Bury St Edmunds, Suffolk
Printed in Great Britain by
Butler and Tanner Ltd, Frome, Somerset

CONTENTS

INTRODUCTION
The Age of Elegance *7*

PART I OUTWARD ELEGANCE
 1 Diet *19*
 2 Exercise *33*
 3 General Health *41*
 4 Sex *59*
 5 Make-up and Skin Care *73*
 6 Hair *93*
 7 Clothes *103*

PART II INWARD ELEGANCE
 8 Personal Style *117*
 9 Spiritual Style *129*
 10 Skill Development *135*

PART III TOTAL ELEGANCE
 11 Homestyle *147*
 12 Workstyle *160*
 13 Lifestyle *175*
 14 Menstyle *189*

AN ELEGANT AFTERWORD *199*

The Elegant Quiz *201*
Useful Addresses *206*

Acknowledgements

Many people contributed their suggestions, knowledge and time to the book, its ideas and information, but special thanks are due to, of course, Pat, Tania, Peta, Kari-Ann, Frances and Sandra and to the women, friends, and others, who generously shared their expertise and experience; and to Life In General for giving it all a framework.

Special thanks also to Jillian Edelstein who took all the photographs; to Kodak who supplied sixty rolls of TRI-X film; to La Cage Imaginaire in Hampstead for their kind permission to photograph there; to Joe's Basement Ltd for developing and contacting the film, and to Max Ferguson for printing.

INTRODUCTION
The Age of Elegance

"When I reached menopause, I realised that as far as Mother Nature was concerned, I was 'not wanted on the voyage'. So I said, 'to hell with you, Mother', and bought an armful of sexy underwear."

If all women faced their middle years with such bravado and confidence, there'd be few tears shed over lost youth and more celebration of what could be, and should be, the best time of a woman's life.

Youth, celebrated in all cultures, looked so attractive when there wasn't much guarantee of a comfortable and enjoyable old age. The consistent bias towards the young was founded on the harshness of life with its primitive medical and scientific knowledge, poor diet and low standard of living, making old age unlikely for most and unpleasant for those who did survive to see it.

Our concept and expectations of "growing older" have changed dramatically in the face of the daily reality of energetic, attractive, dynamic and accomplishing women in business, on the cinema and television screen, in politics and in the high street. The generally high quality of life, medical advances and public awareness of good health and fitness have rolled the idea of "old age" back a decade or two. For the fourteen million women in the UK over forty, mid-life is a turning point, not a turning-off point. They reach for career promotions, not knitting needles; they return to work, they have their first baby, they fill open university courses; they sign up for aerobics, learn Chinese cookery, travel, finally buy their first designer suit, see grown-up children off to college

INTRODUCTION

and think they might join them, take up painting and live in jeans and leggings . . . The "mid-life crisis" is no longer the beginning of the end, but a springboard to a new beginning.

In our great-grandmothers' day it would appear as a chance for a second lifetime. If the first forty years are for awakening to the world, making mistakes and establishing yourself in a career or with a family, the second forty are for enjoying, fulfilling and ripening into a whole being. If you've never had a chance to develop your interests and style fully, this is the time to start. Passing years accumulate rewards that all women inherit and smart women make the most of.

Throw out any idea of "ageing" – with any luck you'll be growing old disgracefully, and gradually, and loving it. Anything over forty is a renaissance, a time of rebirth; a second stage of womanhood which has none of the youthful disadvantages of gaucherie, inexperience, insecurity and uncertainty. True, time costs. No amount of knowledge, vitality and spirit will make fifty-five-year-old skin spring under the touch as it did at twenty-five. It may be painful to admit to yourself that not all of what you wanted to accomplish when you were starting out will be accomplished. You may mourn the gentle creasing and lining of your face, once a blank canvas, now looking definitely lived in – but why shouldn't it? You *have* lived in it, laughed, cried and suffered in it, been joyful, felt pain, wonder and excitement. It *ought* to show. *"Youth's the season made for joys,"* warbled the poet John Gay, *"Life never knows the return of spring."* Maybe, but the warmth, richness and depth of autumn has its own appeal. The past should be remembered with pleasure, not regret, as you move on in changed form to what the second stage of life offers.

◆ ◆ ◆

Renaissance women have one thing youth can't duplicate or compete with – elegance. It's a quality denied to younger women as it depends on the assurance, confidence and inner grace that blossoms with experience in life.

Elegance suffers unjustly from associations with stuffiness, primness or perfection but it is none of these things. Truly elegant women, while appearing stylish and chic, have inner qualities of dignity, generosity and ease. They exude self-

The Age of Elegance

assurance and warmth. Top-to-toe designer outfits aren't elegant, merely expensive. You don't need money to be elegant because its bedrock is strengths money can't buy: confidence, graciousness, compassion, honesty and self-knowledge. Pride, but not vanity. Presence, but not pretentiousness. Assurance without aggression.

Many women discover a new kind of power as they get older. They no longer have to prove themselves to anyone. Their standards are their own. Their self-knowledge and confidence make them equal to any situation. They've sorted out what really matters to them and discarded much of what doesn't matter at all. That subtle aura of being in control, quietly but definitely, is very elegant. The feeling of not having to define or defend yourself, but just be – and be accepted.

All times of change in life have a fragility about them that is unsettling and this time is no exception. Your own physical changes, a divorce or premature death of a spouse, children leaving the nest, moving house or returning to work, reaching a new stage in your relationship with a long-term partner or finding a new partner altogether may make you feel anxious, frightened, resentful, wary. Maturity brings these challenges but also supplies the ammunition to meet them and put them in perspective and put into practice all that wisdom, resilience, resourcefulness and strength the first half of life bequeaths.

◆ ◆ ◆

Still not convinced the Age of Elegance is women's prime time? Consider what riches are on offer:

Self-knowledge: A little honesty means you can afford to be the person you really are, without having to fit anyone else's ideal; this is the time to clarify your desires, sort out interests and as yet unfulfilled dreams and pursue them if you can. You have standards. You know what's open to discussion in the way you live and what's never negotiable.

Power: Career women reach peak performance and top promotion categories in their middle decades, making these productive and satisfying years. The early agonising competitiveness becomes competence. Women who've raised families in these years find they are in new positions of trust and confidence as their children grow into early adulthood themselves. After

INTRODUCTION

years of being at loggerheads with a contrary adolescent, you're not a jailer or a spoilsport any more, but a wise and experienced woman whose love gives credibility to her advice.

Emotional Strength: The great legacy of having lived a bit is the experience and ability to cope with life's knocks and shocks. You've been slapped in the face a few times – fired, divorced, bereaved, betrayed, been given a financial fright, had a great disappointment, and survived it all. You're more thick-skinned, but this toughening is positive and protective.

Personal Style: Twenty years ago you didn't have the confidence to go against the prevailing fashion in clothes, manners or current opinion. Now you've got the moral courage to stick to your convictions whether they set you apart from the crowd or not. You may grow more healthily selfish too, as you refocus attention on to your needs and away from those earlier years when family, job commitments and a partner's needs always seemed to come first.

Health: There's a mountain of information available for older women on maintaining good health and good looks and prolonging their active and involved lives. Regular medical check-ups, a healthy lifestyle, a specific medical treatment for some of the difficulties of growing older, means you can be as fit at fifty as at thirty.

Sexuality: Women are free of the physical anxiety of unwanted pregnancies and the responsibility of looking after a family. Independence and release from these responsibilities is very recharging, sexually. To the outside world you become more interesting. You have a sexual past. You've done nothing but gain over the years in experience, sensuality and understanding. You also know something to which youth is blinded: the difference between sex and love. You've understood how much love isn't physical and have widened as well as deepened the capacity to love and the ability to express it.

Connections: You're not alone. Life-long friends, acquaintances and new branches on the family tree are a connecting, expanding network of your own and your family's history.

Relationships: Long-marrieds can talk more, without the pressing interruptions of family, career decisions and other distractions. Having been through too many problems, good

and bad times, complications and major and minor tragedies together, you've hardly had the time to notice the interdependence, trust and liking that has built up between the two of you. Now it's like lifting the lid off a new relationship. If fate has dealt you a less favourable hand and you're a widow or divorcee, the world is full of potential romance, kindness and passion. Older women have more experience of loving, and know what strengthens a relationship and what destroys it.
Spirituality: Whether or not you give it a name, your soulful traits are honed with maturity. You get wisdom and that major component of elegance, serenity. You may take the fate of the world far more seriously than you did in your younger days, out of concern for your children and grandchildren. You may seek to understand great art, great music, great religion. You look to make a pattern or make sense of the world, seeking to understand something bigger than yourself.

◆ ◆ ◆

Today's renaissance women were young in the 1960s, an era when youthfulness was next to godliness. Everything about the young was worshipped and glorified and reflected in the rapid ascendancy of film and pop stars, the free-flowing, flower-powered clothes, the "swinging" social climate, and the overturning of traditional values. It's not easy to picture the survivors of an era whose slogan was "don't trust anyone over thirty", but here, five famous faces of this youth-centred epoch illustrate the advantage of gaining in years. Pat Knight, Tania Mallet, Frances Meachem, Kari-Ann Moller, and Sandra Paul, stared wide-eyed in miniskirts, white boots and a tonnage of false lashes from dozens of magazine covers and adverts. A sixth, Peta Rogers, dazzled in the season's *haute couture* on the catwalks of London's fashion houses a decade earlier. All six women epitomised the youthful glamour of their time, but were not frozen in it. They've kept the zestful spirit, the interest in looking wonderful and feeling their best, and added the experience of living over the last quarter-century. They have transmuted the freshness of youth into the equally desirable mystery, depth and style that is the allure of the older woman, and throughout this book they'll share their experience and encouragement with women

INTRODUCTION

like yourself who feel a part of this elegant coming of age.

Having begun as models, their early concern was in looking fabulous for the camera or catwalk. Their combined expertise on make-up, clothes and bringing out the best in your appearance is in the first half of this book. Naturally graceful, they've added, through trial, error and instinct, the elegant elements that complete a woman's personality, and explain what and how in the second.

Pat Knight was the face of Max Factor, Gala and Goya make-up and the Teachers whisky girl. Now married, with a son at university, and a passion for the arts, she's returned to modelling and revived earlier ambitions to be a painter.

Although she lives outside London now, she keeps the flat there she once shared with a girlfriend, in their wilder, single days, as a base for visiting friends, working or going to the theatre. Although outward appearance is extremely important to Pat, who's designed as well as modelled clothes, she thinks the prime qualities of elegance are discretion and loyalty. In her clothes elegance is interpreted as "simplicity with dash".

Tania Mallet was labelled the Bond Girl throughout much of her modelling career after colliding with Sean Connery on screen in *Goldfinger*. Her classical features and lean figure and outgoing style made her memorable even in a decade of memorable personalities and faces. A fashion editor remembers her slapping a camel in the face to make it behave during a fashion shoot at Chessington Zoo. Unbothered about signs of ageing, she dubs women at her time of life "the crinklies", in honour of the smile and laugh lines, a testament to having lived a little. *"I don't think there's anything wrong with getting older and showing it,"* she says. Her vision of elegance combines graciousness and discretion with chic style and is most definitely something you grow into. The youth cult is dead, thank God, she says. Now it's time for the grown-ups.

The energetic and effervescent **Frances Meachem** admits she's unfairly always looked ten years younger than her true age, due she says to laughing a lot: *"All your lines go upwards."* A firm believer in seizing the moment and not settling in a rut, she's done some quick changes in her time. She dropped her London life and married a dairy farmer; she

The Age of Elegance

continued modelling until she was thirty-nine then felt she had to do something different before she was forty and opened a successful fashion boutique in the country. Later she sold the business and, with her husband, they now have the farm and a house in London again, plus one in France, and has returned to modelling. Two daughters encourage her to try the latest fashion, from leggings to scarlet lipstick, and she considers this the best time of her life. Part of elegance, she insists, is keeping up with modern trends. *"Memories are lovely, but looking forward is a tonic."*

Kari-Ann Moller – one of Vidal Sassoon's Dolly Birds, she modelled for Mary Quant, had a huge success in London, then fled to a hippie ideal in the country with her artist husband, giving up the King's Road in Chelsea for a renovated, psychedelic-painted garage. Restless again, she returned to London, met and married Chris Jagger, Mick's younger brother, and now lives with him, her four sons and a large dog in an artistically cluttered house in London. She has gone back to modelling and discovered dance. Sitting by the fireside, her long hair loose, and dressed in brilliantly coloured flowing clothes, she looks like a beautiful witch. Naturally elegant, poised and unselfconscious, she admires elegance, not as contrived perfection, but likens it to an old building, stylish and comfortable in its surroundings.

Sandra Paul is a former supermodel, occasional journalist and mother of three, now married to a Westminster politician. Sensitivity, she says, is one ingredient of elegance. Unpretentious and understanding of the difficulties women face coming to terms with their changing selves, she claims one benefit of gaining in years is that you can afford to be yourself and lose *"that terrible self-consciousness of youth"*.

Peta Rogers was a top house model at London fashion houses, including Hardy Amies where the clients she modelled for were occasionally royalty, both real (Princess Marina, Princess, now Queen, Elizabeth) and reel (Vivien Leigh). She worked in public relations, as a fashion commentator, and was the fashion editor of a major woman's magazine. Now in her seventies she's lost none of the grace, suppleness and high style that fuelled her on the runways. Time brings

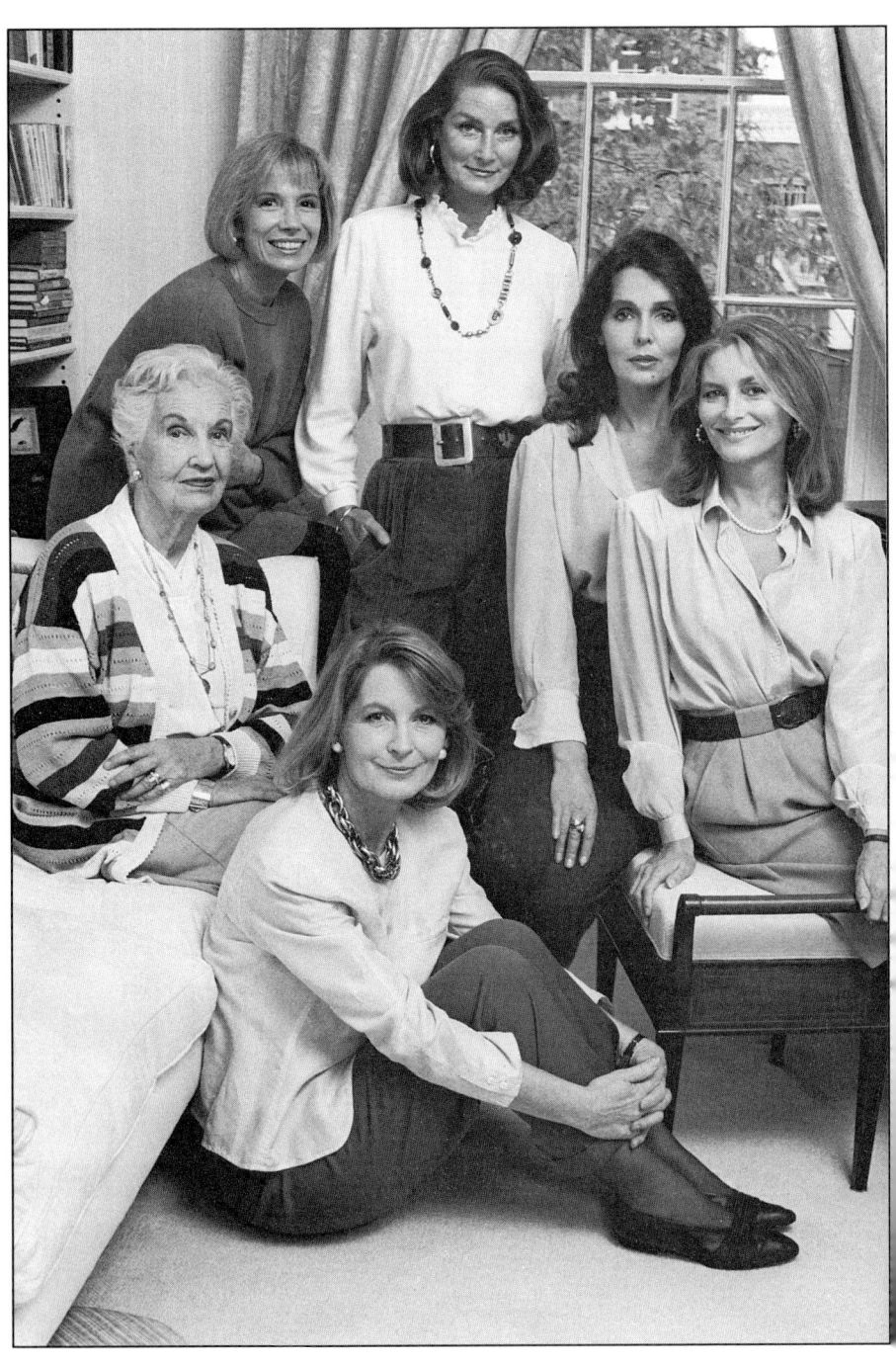

Clockwise from left: Peta Rogers, Frances Meachem, Tania Mallet, Kari-Ann Moller and Pat Knight. Seated in front, Sandra Paul.

The Age of Elegance

compensations, she says. *"You have a serenity that's lacking when you're young, and a greater awareness of other people. The young are always trying to be something they're not. It's only later you accept yourself and can afford to reach out to other people. That genuine interest and warmth towards others is very elegant."*

All six women have an elegance which touches every area of life – appearance and personal chic, relationships in and out of the home, work, play and their own self-image.

Like kindness, elegance costs nothing but enhances life a great deal. The following chapters reveal how you too can have it, and how it can change and enhance your life.

An elegant checklist

The *OED* defines elegance as "refined grace of form", "tastefulness of adornment", "simplicity and effectiveness".

Elegance is most often seen by comparison. Everything about the Regency period, for example, its architecture, fashion and furniture, was elegant in a way the Victorian era was not. Likewise, a simple well-cut shift dress may be more elegant than a bespangled, be-bowed, frilled and fluttery one. Elegance always looks effortless.

You can measure your own elegance quotient against the following:

Elegant	Inelegant
A ten-year-old Harris tweed jacket	A ten-minute-old imitation leather bomber
Wool, cotton, silk	Plastic, vinyl, rubber
Well-cut jeans	Ripped jeans
Court pumps	White stilettos
Stockings	Pop socks
A man's watch	A Mickey Mouse watch
Real jewellery	Loads of fake or cheap jewellery, especially gold chains
Fresh flowers	One too many bowls of pot pourri
Keeping a friend's painful secret	Popping down the pub to let the regulars know what's going on
Having a discreet affair	Calling the tabloids if you've seen his picture in the paper

PART I

OUTWARD ELEGANCE

No one of any age, whether six or sixty, faces life with enjoyment and enthusiasm if they are in poor health, look shabby and feel low. The older you are the more difficult it is for a body to fight off the ill effects of physical excesses, sickness or a sedentary lifestyle. Gone are the days when your body bounced back from too much food and drink and you had the stamina to go without sleep, living on excitement. Years of thoughtless indulgences and, frankly, gravity, often give women a salutary shock when they stand in front of a full-length mirror after the bath or in a department store fitting-room and see someone else's body *reflected back. Surely that can't be me, they say? I've always had firm thighs and a flat tum. Alas, one of the changes in later life is shifting shape, as fatty tissue gathers around abdomen and thighs, transforming your traditional hour-glass shape into the common pear shape. Weak stomach muscles, overeating and irregular exercise exaggerate the pear. Seeing it for the first time, said a woman despairingly, is like walking into your favourite room and seeing all the wallpaper hanging down.*

But inside the news is good: your heart still beats seventy-two times a minute, lung capacity tapers off only gradually — unless you smoke, in which case you have only half the lung capacity of non-smokers to begin with — the joints are still reasonably elastic and all these bits and pieces should see you through if you keep them well-tuned. Far from being too late to meddle with nature, it's just the time for an overhaul. Assuming you have no major health problems you can mop up the mistakes of the first forty years and fine tune and reinvent yourself for the next forty. No one is going to live out their years healthily and elegantly if they abuse the basic equipment, inside and out. Maintaining a healthy body in good repair is not just aesthetically pleasing; it prolongs your life and ensures you have the stamina and vitality to enjoy it. You know this is leading up to a lecture about diet and exercise, but don't say you've heard it all before. Put down that biscuit and listen. Some stories get better with the telling.

1 ◆ *Diet*

It's a rare woman who hasn't been overweight at some time in her life – baby fat, adolescent puppy fat, post-natal poundage, middle-age spread: some women have had it all. You're old enough to be free of the thinner-than-thou philosophy that tyrannises women from their teens, and aim for fitness, strength and wellness now, rather than tiny measurements. Having said that, most women admit to being a few pounds over their ideal weight. Many are quite a few over, trying to lose that stone that just won't budge, usually in desperate crash dieting before a holiday or family wedding. Some women find they no longer shed excess pounds as easily as they once did in their salad days – *"I'm into my dessert days now,"* says one, *"and it shows."* A few have been overweight for so long they've given up hope of ever taking it off and regaining their slim selves. Thinness, slimness, is so important to women because being fat is a social crime.

Fat is a four-letter word in society. Some of the antipathy is based on health grounds – we know obese people are at greater risk from coronary disease and complications associated with other ailments such as respiratory disease, diabetes and high blood pressure. But much of the prejudice against fat is social.

Generally speaking, fat people have a more difficult time socially and professionally, and it takes a great personality or explosive talent to overcome the physical liability. It's not only the look of wobbly thighs or a large bottom drooping out of a swimsuit that offends sensibilities. Fat is a symbol of poor self-control, weakness, low self-esteem, even less intelligence. When a very overweight woman walks into a room, it's unlikely the men will flash a look of interest and desire at the newcomer; the slimmest, smartest women will turn away also: she is not "one of us".

Obviously no woman is the sum total of her weight on the scales, but there is no scale or public measure which registers her talents, skills, loyalty, humour and intellect. Outsiders often don't make the effort to get past the fat barrier and overweight women know it. A woman who is self-conscious, uncomfortable and unhappy about her weight will be less assertive in social situations. Feelings of self-worth may be at low ebb. Expectations are low. When women are, or feel, fat, they don't expect to be flirted with, arouse male interest at a dinner party, catch the eye of the new vice-president as a candidate for promotion, be admired by other women or their daughters' friends. They're treated with less deference and consideration than their slimmer sisters at the make-up counter, in a dress boutique, or at the hairdressers. They get less of a hearing at the doctor's, the lawyer's or the complaints department of any organisations. Society's message is very clear: if you don't care enough about yourself to look good, we won't care about you either. If you think you're not worth the effort of guarding your health, we'll take your word for it: you're not worth it. It doesn't take much of that sort of treatment before a woman starts to believe, and accept, it.

Sometimes the way a woman looks in reality is quite different from her own inner image of herself. Teenage anorexics insist they are "fat" even when they plainly see ribs, hip-bones and knee joints protruding. At the other end of the scale, it may be a "truth" in your family that you've always had a "lovely figure" or "wonderful legs", without noticing or taking in how time has spread the bottom out, widened the hips or produced a sag here and there. Or, you may have triumphed and slimmed down to size ten, but on days when you feel under the weather or hate what you're wearing, you feel "fat".

Being deeply unhappy with your physical appearance undermines your relationships, withers your sex life, social life, and holds you back from exploring new opportunities in new surroundings, because it eats away at your confidence. You can't appear happily on the beach if you're agonising over a

Diet

tummy bulge; you won't feel powerful going for a job interview with a suit jacket straining at the armpits.

Every woman, even the slimmest, knows these feelings of doubt and self-disgust, when something about her dress or feelings or attitude that day makes it a "fat day", even though the scales register the same as yesterday. You feel more like hiding away than job hunting or meeting someone new. If every day is a "fat day" it's time to do something about it.

Women should consult a doctor or well woman clinic where they may be recommended to see a dietician before embarking on a serious weight loss regime if they are substantially overweight. Those who struggle with a stone or two, losing some, gaining some, in a continual seesaw, need to revamp their eating habits more than diet. One of the tragedies of dieting is that once it all comes off, it usually all goes back on again just being in the same room as chocolate cake. That's why a diet is a good kickstart to a healthy eating pattern but a poor mode to live by. Nobody can exist on lettuce leaves and cottage cheese for ever in a world full of walnut whips and Italian bread. A diet is only the beginning of a change in attitude to eating, a change that should enable you to slim down without dampening all enjoyment of food. Most dieters set themselves impossible goals and targets that are guaranteed to fail. Life is too short to never have another plate of hot buttered toast or slice of fudgy cake, but your life may be very and unnecessarily short if you make it a habit to stuff on them regularly.

Because being overweight so weakens self-esteem and stops women projecting their best selves, it can never be elegant. However there are some large – not fat – women, who refuse to be bullied by *Vogue* or any arbiters of fashion and whose positive presence, great confidence and unabashed ease at their appearance projects an elegant style. In fact, says Sandra Paul, a bit of extra flesh often suits mature women. *"Being overweight isn't elegant, but if you're in proportion, a bit over can be extremely becoming. You don't look as lined and your shoulders look wonderful in evening dress."*

Despite her comforting words, it's estimated that at any

one time, half the female population is on a slimming regime. The other half have given up today but vow to start again tomorrow.

Before you consider any diet, it's most important to know clearly *why* you want to lose weight. It must be for your own good health, because looking wonderful boosts your confidence and self-esteem and makes you more capable and assertive in facing the challenges of the day. And because you might get stranded in a snowstorm with Harrison Ford. A diet has first and foremost got to be for you, not to please your mother or children solely, or to impress a friend. The pleasure and approval of your nearest and dearest is a nice bonus, but not the goal. When you're doing it for yourself first, when the inspiration, drive and determination is from you and for you, you're more likely to make a success of any diet. At your age you've probably read several thousand words on diets, so you already know that your body needs the right fuel to function with maximum ability and pleasure, physically and mentally. It will keep going on chips and fags, but not for long. Just as the wrong fuel clogs up car and machine engines, so your body will keep working, but sluggishly and rebelliously. The rebellion may take the shape of excess weight, or greyish, dull skin that constantly breaks out in blemishes, or, that curse of the bikini set, cellulite. Cellulite, which gives skin an unattractive, dimpled, "orange peel" look is believed to be caused by fluid trapped in fatty tissues because of poor circulation and diet. Most cellulite-battling diets include a detoxifying diet which ban caffeine, tobacco, alcohol, red meat and dairy products, and a vigorous skin-toning programme of massages and body scrubs.

Psychological health is also affected by what you eat. Depression, apathy, and tiredness can be caused by an imbalanced diet, usually one too heavy in refined sugars and stodge. The opposite is also true: a really fit, well-nourished body withstands the assaults of illness and stress much better than a nutritionally run-down one.

Pat Knight revamped her diet not to lose weight but to recapture her ebbing vitality. *"A couple of years ago I was convinced I had the yuppie flu,"* she explains. *"I was tired and depressed all the time. I had no energy and felt dreadful. A naturopath recommended a vegetarian raw food diet and though I was sceptical and it sounded peculiar I was ready to try anything."*

For four months she stuck to raw vegetables and fruit and *"felt marvellous. All my energy returned."*

Life being full of temptations for dieters, however, she found four months of rigid dieting enough. *"One day we were in Stratford and everyone was having smoked salmon. I just couldn't stand it any longer, so I had a plateful and buckets of potato salad – and was sick afterwards of course. Now I've modified my diet to include a lot of raw food but make it more workable for everyday living. The experience got me interested in diet and I did a lot of investigating before creating one that suits me."* The ideal dinner she outlines wouldn't satisfy a meat, potatoes and pudding woman, but many dieters would find Pat's "plate of stuff" generous and satisfying. On a large platter she piles up: brown rice or jacket potato, avocado, cashew nuts, broccoli or mange tout, red pepper, half a pear, lettuce or radicchio, sunflower and sesame seeds. The "stuff" is sprinkled with a home-made dressing of cider vinegar, dry mustard, honey and sunflower oil. *"Delicious,"* she says. Women longing to smother some butter or sour cream on that jacket potato probably won't enjoy Pat's breakfast substitute of mineral water instead of milk on her muesli.

But that really is the point about dieting and why so few women can stick to one regime for very long. Unless it's full of foods you like to eat and can easily prepare, it's too easy to give up. The search for a diet that lets you eat all the yummy things you crave, all the time, is one reason why a never-ending succession of diets come and go out of fashion. We've all tried the Scarsdale diet, Weight Watchers, the Pritikin, the Beverly Hills, the Cambridge, the F-plan – but at the end of the day it comes down to how many calories you swallow. It's too simple to be true: eat more calories than your body burns up, you'll get fat. Eat fewer, you'll get thin.

Starvation, crash diets, and diet pills were, are and always will be out of fashion for anyone pursuing health or with a grain of common sense.

An average woman will keep going on 2,000 calories a day, although a sedentary woman, or an older woman who has given up regular exercise, may burn fewer. To take weight off, a woman must stick to 1,000–1,200 calories a day, spread out over three to five meals. Gorging a day's worth of calories in one go – a legacy from our caveman ancestors – spurs your body to release insulin, which will turn most of your calorific intake into stored fat. Eating several small meals throughout the day actually reduces the release of insulin and prevents fat being stored.

Some sacrifices hardly qualify as suffering: switching from whole milk to skimmed, from butter to low fat spread, and grilling rather than frying. But no amount of wishful thinking will make cheese, unless it's the very low fat variety, a good diet food: it's almost as loaded with calories as chocolate. Four ounces of delicious Cheddar has 250 calories while bland old cottage cheese only 110. *One* ounce of rich creamy Gouda has 100. The same blatant unfairness extends to "healthy" foods like cereals. Muesli, so virtuous to eat, delivers 300 calories in a four-ounce serving compared with cornflakes' modest 90. No wonder dieters get cross and crabby. To make up for it slightly, some foods have virtually no calories at all – cucumber, tomatoes, celery and red peppers can be eaten literally until you can't eat any more. Because you can't judge the calorific impact of food by looking at it, weighing it or wishing it were something different, all dieters need a good calorie counter if on a weight loss diet. Calorie counters are plentiful and inexpensive in bookshops and often supermarket check-outs where they make frightening reading in the line-up, adding up all the calories in your trolley.

If the stress of going on a diet is enough and you can't be bothered totting up every crumb and morsel, be guided by lean and disciplined Tania Mallet who, like all the models in this book, has kept to the slim regime of her early days and is still "camera ready" attractive.

"As a rule of thumb, fat makes you fat," says Tania, *"so cut it down and out and you'll be all right. I don't eat meat because it's high in fat, even though it was once a staple in*

diets; I love pasta and potatoes, which used to be forbidden, but savouries are my downfall. I love cheese and I do like a drink. You do have to be sensible but you can't take all the enjoyment out of life. You have to find a balance."

Part of the balance is knowing the difference between good fat and bad fat. True, when you're looking in the mirror there is only bad fat, but to your body there is a good kind too, a kind it needs in tiny quantities for healthy bones and teeth. Many women eat too much of both kinds of fats – when your diet is half fat, so will you be. The visible fats like butter and cream are easy to see and cut out but there is fat in almost everything and much of it is hidden until it shows up around your waistline. Red meat and poultry skin contain high quantities of fat, as do biscuits, whole milk, pastry and cakes while eggs are high in cholesterol, a fat that is not only physically enlarging, but dangerous, as it is believed to clog up arteries and lead to heart disease. But fatty-fish such as salmon and mackerel contain fish oils which are beneficial to your heart. Every new step forward in research and discovery brings a barrage of conflicting opinions, but generally it is accepted that saturated fats increase cholesterol levels in the blood, poly-unsaturated fats actually reduce cholesterol levels, while mono-unsaturates provide vitamins A, D, E and K as well as some fatty acids which are essential to good health.

The bad fats to avoid in large quantities are the saturated fats which come mainly from animals: milk, cheese, butter, lard and meat. If you do regularly eat meat, reduce the fat content by trimming of all the visible fat and skim the fat off stews and casseroles. Animal fat is also widely used for baking and much frying is done with lard. Switching from these animal saturates to vegetable mono- or poly-unsaturates such as olive oil, and using butter substitutes made with sunflower, safflower, corn or soya bean oil reduces not only cholesterol levels but calorie levels too. When cooking, skimmed milk is an undetectable substitute for fatty whole milk, and recipes that cry out for cream as a *coup de grâce* can be elegantly finished off with low fat yoghurt instead.

Next to fat, sugar is the enemy for most dieters and all

women pursuing a healthier lifestyle. Health-faddists used to feel noble spooning down honey until told it's just sugar in another form. Refined sugar is the problem, the kind that's packed into candy and biscuits. Sucrose, as opposed to the more slowly metabolising fructose found in fruits, does give you a quick fix (and adds weight and a craving for more) but carbohydrates and fruit will give you more staying power. Many women learn to like and even prefer the taste of artificial sweeteners in tea or coffee; others discover that food has been "oversweetened" for years and find the natural sweetness of raisins, apricots and other rich fruits in baking means they need to use next to no sugar.

One drawback of dieting in mid-life is that metabolism, the body's ability to burn up calories, is slowing down, making it more difficult to shed weight. That extra ten pounds you put on every winter and dropped every spring may cling obstinately now. On the plus side, however, older women experience a change in appetite and many of the rich foods they once enjoyed now seem sickening, not satisfying. Says Sandra Paul, *"I've been conditioned all my life not to eat rich things and now I find I can't. They make me ill. I eat what feels comfortable, although I do have some rules for myself like bread* or *potatoes and pudding* or *cheese, but not both, at dinner, but rich and greasy foods I now loathe."*

Some women find a "food attitude" that is an expression and extension of their life philosophy, making it somewhat easier to stick to. Kari-Ann Moller, attuned to the alternative lifestyles of the New Age, has a truckload of organic vegetables delivered every week from the country to her London house. *"Even the marmalade in the cupboard is organic,"* she enthuses. *"Every time I say that word, my sons roll their eyes and cringe! We're very health conscious in this house but we don't deprive ourselves – we have biscuits and ice cream occasionally, but it's always very good quality ice cream, natural ingredients and all that."*

It's the "all that" that defeats dieters. Too many diet systems call for operational and pre-planning control that rivals the army. Shopping for the right food, adding up the calories, planning menus, eating up the last left-overs before you even begin . . . Whatever kind of diet you embark on it must fit your lifestyle and cause minimum upheaval and inconvenience. There's no point spending hours preparing strange foodstuffs in rigid proportions that won't travel outside your own kitchen. You may have to diet, but you also have to live. One hostess bemoaned the time the whole world seemed to be following Weight Watchers: *"It was hell at dinner parties; everybody pushing into the kitchen to measure their portions of meat or fish down to the last quarter-ounce. I gave up inviting some people."*

Likewise, the Pritikin diet was abandoned by a woman who felt ridiculous bringing bags of "birdseed" as she called the Pritikin staple mix of nuts, seeds and raisins, to other people's houses.

Extremes may be effective for a week or two but after that you'll slip into old habits. What's wanted is not a diet but an approach to eating that becomes an ingrained style, as unremarkable as brushing your teeth. "I'd like to reach the point," confessed a lifelong dieter, "where having a second helping of pudding isn't an either/or, should I, shouldn't I debate. I'd like it to be not on, ever, so I don't have to think about it." A change in eating habits takes time to establish itself, and lifelong dieters tend to be impatient as well as greedy, but it is worth making the effort. Just because it is so hard to alter a lifetime of unhealthy overeating, it's doubly unfair that a lot of diet sabotage comes from a woman's loved ones.

Once you've made up your mind that you simply cannot be fifty, sixty, seventy, without losing that extra stone and coming down a dress size:

◆ **Don't** listen to your husband/lover/mother who loves you just the way you are. If you don't love you, change you.

◆ **Don't** listen to the friend who jollies you into agreeing "we're too old to worry about that now. We don't have to bother." Bother.

And, once you're launched:

◆ **Don't** tidy up left-over food, the last slice of bread, the last mouthful of pie, just because it's there or won't fit in the fridge. Give it to your friend, she's not bothered.

◆ **Don't** buy cream as a treat for coffee, then pour it over pie or cake to use it up "before it goes off". Let it go off, or you'll be off.

◆ **Don't** eat when doing something else, like watching telly or reading.

◆ **Don't** eat bread rolls in restaurants before the main meal.

◆ **Don't** scoff biscuits while waiting for the kettle to boil.

◆ **Don't** eat in a hurry. It's shocking how much food you can shovel in without tasting it.

◆ **Don't** pick at food between meals. Give your stomach a chance to get rid of a meal and be empty before you load it up again. Snacking and nibbling means you never stop thinking about food and never give yourself a break from it. To be always fretting and feeding is very stressful.

◆ Never use laxatives or emetics to get rid of over-indulgences.

It's always easier to overeat when you're tired, stressed, fed up and bored and it's especially easy for women since they're usually the food preparers in the household, handling temptation hourly. Stress must have an outlet and it's socially more acceptable for women to be seen with an ice cream or bun in their hand than a large gin.

Dieting is slow, tedious work so don't be too hard on yourself. Food is delicious, one of life's true pleasures. It serves no purpose to cut yourself off from all treats and everyone overindulges sometimes, so shove away the guilt. Life isn't so full of pleasure that you have to turn down every temptation that comes your way, including edible ones. Stick to a basically healthy, well-planned diet, low in fat, high in fibre, with something from all food groups daily: milk and milk products (dairy), fresh fruit and vegetables (greens), meat, fish and eggs (proteins) and wholegrains (carbohydrates), and you can have your bit of cake and eat it too, once in a while, without a troubled conscience.

◆ ◆ ◆

Diet

You don't really need to be reminded but:

Reasonable Breakfast: Half a grapefruit, slice of wholemeal toast, or bowl of cereal; varying with slice of toast and boiled or poached egg.

Unreasonable Breakfast: Chocolate croissant; cereal with cream; two slices buttered toast with marmalade.

Reasonable Lunch: Tuna salad on wholemeal bread, yoghourt or fresh fruit.

Unreasonable Lunch: Beefburger and chips, knickerbocker glory.

Reasonable Dinner: Grilled fish or chicken, green salad, jacket potato, fruit salad with frozen yoghurt.

Extremely Unreasonable Dinner: Breaded veal, scalloped potatoes, buttered roll, apple crumble with custard or cream.

And look at what else you already know about slimline eating: you can eat apples, beans, lettuce, cucumber, tomatoes, all citrus fruits, pineapple, courgettes and melons. But *not* canned fruit in syrup, lima beans, chick peas, peas, sweetcorn or dried fruits, although some dried fruit such as apricots are a good source of calcium. Likewise you don't need to be told that chicken, lean beef, fish and shellfish are healthy additions to a diet, while battered fish, bacon, sausages, salami and stews aren't for slimmers, and should be eaten in moderation even if you're not slimming.

Many nutritionists declare that a well-balanced diet provides all the vitamins a body needs, yet more vitamin supplements are sold over the counter than any other product, including analgesics.

Whether it's an indication we deliberately choose our food poorly or whether we feel something is more likely to be effective if we pay for it, is open to debate. It is true that whatever good intentions we have when choosing and cooking food we don't always live up to the ideal of little fat, lots of fibre, and steaming and grilling rather than boiling and frying. A great many of us eat too much refined and overprocessed food. A multivitamin supplement does correct any imbalances and it won't hurt whatever else you put into your body that day.

Some people are natural candidates for vitamin supplements: junk-food addicts who eat too much overprocessed rubbish, pregnant and breastfeeding women, elderly people who've stopped having regular meals or skip meals, those recovering from illness and heavy drinkers and smokers whose addiction inhibits the absorption of vitamins from their food. A multivitamin is the most common "all-rounder" but many women take individual extras, such as vitamin C to ward off colds, extra calcium to strengthen bones and vitamin B for stress.

It's not enough just to swallow a supplement. What you mix with it can affect its potency and effectiveness. For example, smoking increases the amount of stomach acid which undermines digestion, robbing the body of vitamins C and B. Foods that include drugs, like caffeine and tannin in coffee and tea, also make it difficult for the body to absorb minerals and vitamins. Some dieticians recommend either not drinking tea or coffee with a meal or switching to decaffeinated. Without vitamin C you may be anaemic because of iron deficiency; one of vitamin C's functions is to help the body store iron. Vitamins A, D and E are stored by the body but the C and B groups are water-soluble and have to be replenished every day. As appetite and preferences change with age, you may feel now is the time for an additional boost from vitamins. The following chart outlines what some of the more common nutrients do. Make sure you never exceed the recommended dose.

Vitamin/Mineral	Source	Action
Vitamin A	eggs, spinach, fish oils, dairy products	healthy hair and nails
B1 (thiamine)	wholemeal bread, nuts, brown rice	turns carbohydrates to energy
B2 (riboflavin)	wholegrains, cheese, red meat	converts fats, sugars and protein to energy
B6	wholegrains, eggs, liver, vegetables	healthy skin and hair and makes anti-stress hormones
B12	dairy products, red meat	healthy blood and tissue
Vitamin C	citrus fruits and fresh vegetables	healthy teeth, gums and bones, and boosts body's immune system
Vitamin D	oily fish, sunshine	promotes calcium for bones

Diet

Vitamin/Mineral	Source	Action
Vitamin E	green vegetables, eggs, vegetable oils	boosts circulatory system, makes essential fatty acids
Calcium	dairy products, sardines (whole), apricot, tofu	healthy bones and teeth, and may help stave off osteoporosis
Selenium	fish, grains, cereal	makes antibodies

◆ ◆ ◆

In addition to these familiar vitamins and supplements, many women swear by the improving effects of "alternative" supplements such as oil of evening primrose, royal jelly and oriental ginseng. Evening primrose oil is taken by many women to relieve premenstrual symptoms but even in later life they find it a healing and restorative addition to their diets. Kari-Ann Moller used to take royal jelly regularly but gave it up when she became convinced its collection from the hives did more harm than the jelly did good to her skin and general air of youthfulness. Ginseng has a romantic lure of its own, long touted as promoting sexual stamina, and as a general tonic for well-being and energy. Although there is no definitive scientific proof that these supplements do what their devotees claim, if you feel happy, well-maintained and positive in taking them, their addition to your diet is invaluable.

Dieting is never easy and always feels unfair. Some dieters use props to help them through the early days: a backview of themselves on the beach last summer pasted on the fridge door, sayings "eat to live, not live to eat" on the corkboard. Some use bribes, like buying a gorgeous new dress in a size too small and keeping it hanging out in a room where it's a constant and tantalising reminder of your goal. In addition to reducing the flesh, diets tend to reduce tempers and patience too. Indulge yourself with a few treats like fresh flowers, expensive make-up, the new bestseller, those heavily glossy European fashion magazines which are too pricey for regular consumption, perfume – something that lessens the feeling of deprivation.

Spreading the good word won't make you popular either. Convincing a partner or family that there is a healthy, tasty

OUTWARD ELEGANCE

life after fish-fingers and chips is not for the faint-hearted, and it's a strong woman who can defend herself against inner temptation and outside hostility. But she will be a fitter, healthier and more elegant woman because of it.

Dieting Checklist
♦ An elegant dieter uses as many different and unusual vegetables as she can find in her dishes to keep boredom at bay. These include celeriac, mange tout, kohlrabi, okra and squash. She does the same with fruits: tamarillo, kumquat, mango, kiwi and star fruit are infinitely more interesting than oranges and apples.
♦ An elegant dieter does not eat all the chocolate mousse intended for the evening's company and blame its disappearance on the dog.

2 ♦ *Exercise*

Regular exercise must be as natural a part of a woman's everyday routine as brushing her hair or cleaning her teeth. Its benefits are at least as great. Just as you wouldn't dream of setting off for the day unwashed and unkempt, so you shouldn't miss the vital routine that trims, tones and rejuvenates the body. Exercise awakens and calms the mind, builds up resistance to stress and emotional trauma, defeats lethargy, oils the joints and primes the muscles, and infuses you with energy.

What's more, the need for exercise increases with the years. Loss of flexibility and mobility is the curse of growing older. Imagine an "old woman". Is your mental image bent and crooked, the woman stooped in the hunched and humped posture of "old age"? She needn't be. Exercise is preventative medicine against the stiffening of joints and the bone-thinning disease osteoporosis which causes brittle bones and the stereotypical "dowager's hump" of old age. Women as young as fifty can show signs of it. Beautifully dressed, poised, clever, charming, they can never be elegant with tense, rounded shoulders and neck and stiff movements. This poor posture pushes your belly out too, giving a woman that "squashed down" look familiar in the elderly. Good posture, flexibility, sitting and standing tall, can easily take years off a woman's age.

Women who haven't exercised for years cling to the heresy that it's too late to start now. Anyone of any age can be fit; but fit doesn't mean running an eight-minute mile or defeating a younger opponent at squash. Real fitness is a combination of stamina, suppleness, strength and agility. Natural skill comes in there somewhere, but that determines perhaps just how important or enjoyable an activity is, not how fit you are.

Anyone who exercises regularly knows that optimism and confidence, as well as energy, rise after a workout. Even better, like a gift from the gods, it improves your sex life. Almost half the women interviewed in an American study said their sex lives were more active since they started exercising. Obviously feeling proud of their bodies and being full of energy gave them confidence and freedom in the bedroom. Nothing is worse than going away for a romantic weekend and wondering if your knee cartilage is really going to stand up to it.

Exercise also works wonders for depression. Intense physical activity releases endorphins in the body, the so-called "happy hormones" which flood you with feelings of wellbeing and contentment. It's why people who exercise regularly get "addicted" to it, feeling rough and low if they're forced to miss a day or two.

Most women approach exercise with rather the same mixed feelings as they approach dieting. Many have made sporadic attempts to find and stick to an exercise programme and have abandoned it as readily. At the back of women's cupboards throughout the nation are discarded exercise clothes, comprising a potted fashion history of exercise over the last decade or two. There are the tennis whites, the lime-green aerobics workout suit, the unflattering Speedo swimsuit and goggles, the trainers and racket from when squash was ultra-fashionable, the cushioned jogging shoes. Now you've been through the gamut of things you don't like, it's time to settle into an exercise routine you do like, that gives you pleasure, that does the good physical work it's designed to do and that you can stick to for life. The whole point of exercise is to improve your present and take out a little insurance on your future, not to see how much you can suffer. Unless you've exercised consistently over the past decade the harsher, more demanding physical workouts are best left to the younger and more dedicated. Fast-paced aerobics and jogging are too punishing on joints and lungs for a novice.

Fragile ligaments and unstretched muscles deserve a little

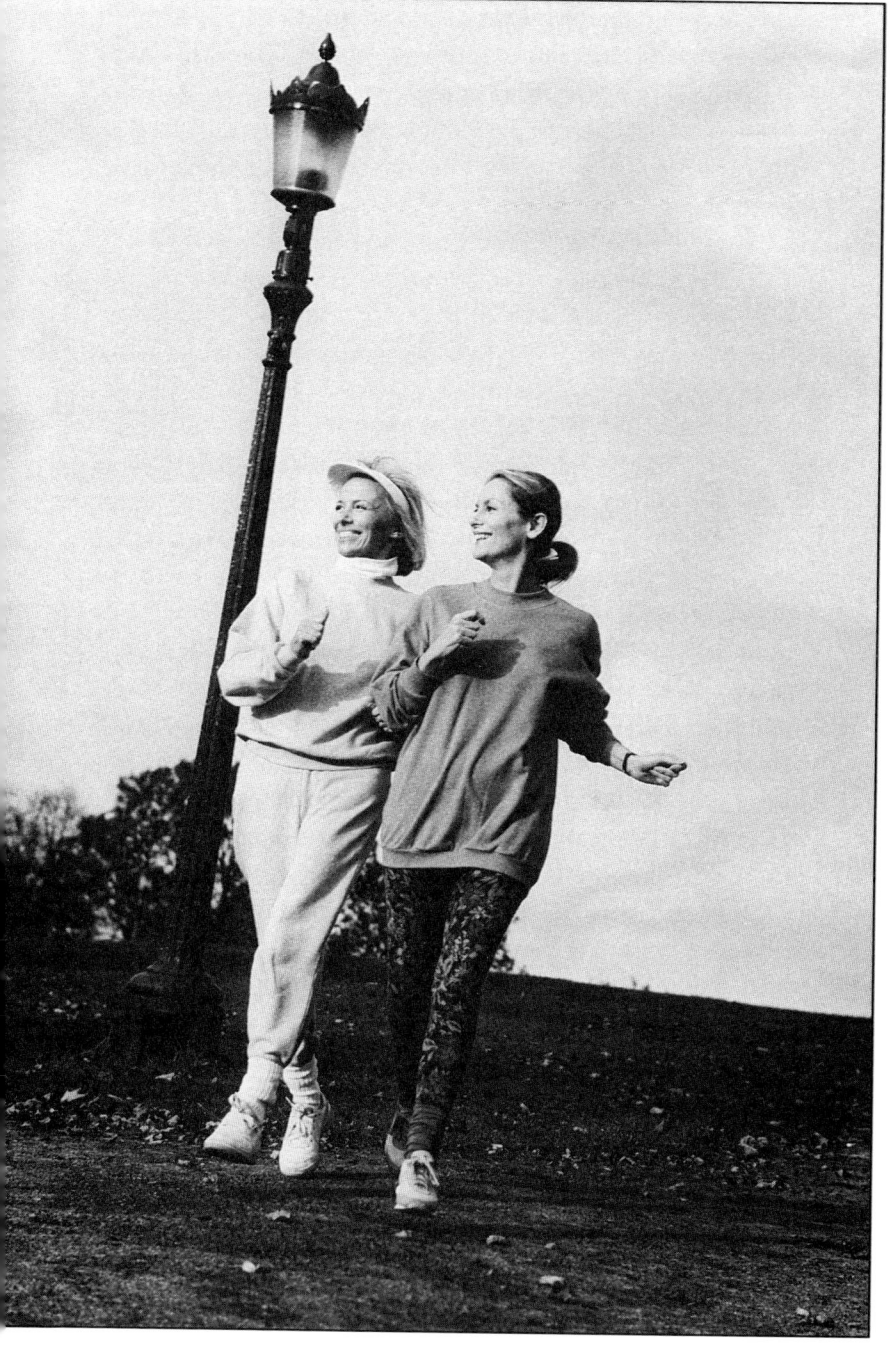

cushioning, which is why swimming is an ideal activity. In addition to using all the muscles in the body, it aids co-ordination, and there is the soothing, healing aspect of spending time in the water. Water is comforting, and the physical buoyancy is echoed by emotional buoyancy too. Peta Rogers, who moves with the grace and ease of a woman half her seventy-plus years, begins each day with eight laps of the pool. *"It's part of my daily routine, I hardly think of it as exercising,"* she says. *"I'm lucky I like it; it makes me feel really* well, *and it's not a chore."*

Not every woman is fortunate enough to have ready access to a pool year round, but everyone has access to roads and parks to walk. A brisk half-hour every day raises the heart rate, increases circulation and keeps the limbs springy. Best of all, after the initial investment of comfortable shoes, walking is free and available every day of the year. Nor is it chained to a club or recreation centre's timetable. Some women like to pull on a jogging suit and walking shoes before breakfast, take their brisk and determined turn around the common and come back to bath, breakfast and a fresh new day. Others prefer a revitalising evening walk that refreshes them enough mentally to feel good but tires them physically to make sleep come easily. A committed walker admitted she started her evening quickstep to try and defeat persistent insomnia, a common problem in later life (see page 49). Even more than the physically tiring, she said, the mental and emotional unwinding made sleep possible for the first time in years.

When these women talk about walking they are not describing a stroll or a meander through the shops. However gently you start, and it should be gentle if this is your first exercise since tights took over from stockings and suspenders, you're building up to a fast walking pace, just at the point before breaking into a jog. Your heart rate should be up, you should feel warm, perspiring slightly but not panting or strained. Of course as you gradually get fit and your body tone improves, the amount your heart rate increases will reduce, and you will be able to stride out longer and stronger. If you are really out of condition it is advisable to consult your doctor before you start any exercise regime.

Exercise

Although "a walk" sounds such a common and unexciting exercise compared with high impact aerobics or water-polo, as exercise it deserves to be taken seriously. In addition to the right shoes, you should always wear light, comfortable clothing, preferably in layers in cooler weather so you can peel them off as your body temperature rises with exertion. Decent waterproof clothing and headgear is also a must so that inclement weather won't give you an excuse to stay in and eat biscuits by the telly. A proper waterproof with zipped pockets to hold your door key and identification is ideal. As this is exercise time, not shopping or browsing time, you won't need a handbag or heavy shoulderbag to weigh you down and distort your posture as you "walk out". You can go shopping after you exercise. Hands and arms need to be free to fall into the natural swing motion as you walk with shoulders back and down and chin up. Stretch your spine up. Breathe deeply from time to time to expand your lungs. Inhale as deeply as possible, feeling your diaphragm lift and midrift expand and open up to the rush of air. Although you must choose the best time for you, immediately after a meal is not a good idea, as is any exercising on a full stomach. An empty stomach isn't good either: if you go first thing in the morning as many joggers and runners do, have an orange, some juice and a plain biscuit to give yourself something to go on.

Each woman knows her home terrain best and those lucky enough to be close to a park or common will take their best walks there. Exercise some common sense as well as your muscles and don't choose a route that will take you through heavy traffic where the damage of breathing in the car and lorry fumes will undo any benefits. Veteran walkers say that choosing an emotionally satisfying route, such as one through parkland or heath where greenery, plants and wild flowers and bird and animal life are part of your routine, makes the whole process more satisfying. One woman who found it difficult to keep her impetus to get outside at seven every morning, even though she loved the crispness and quiet of the morning air and the vitality the walk gave her, bought a dog to spur her on. *"He has to go out,"* she says, *"so I have to go with him. I call him my personal trainer."*

If imposing routine and discipline on yourself is too much of a burden, join a class and be cajoled, bullied and inspired into fitness by like-minded people. Although many groups are heavily weighted towards tough aerobics or fast-moving competitive games like netball and badminton, there are a clutch of strength-and-movement classes about if you root around in your area. The best known is yoga, a staple of adult evening classes and a perfect exercise programme for older women with its emphasis on slow, precise but flowing movements. There is no speed, pressure or strain as participants work towards relaxation of both body and mind. Unfortunately many women still connect yoga with a turbaned mystic standing on his head, legs knotted in an impossible position, breathing through one nostril. The positions for long-time practitioners of yoga may hold such challenges but most women find they are taught controlled and relaxed breathing, stretching and flexing exercises, and rapidly become more supple, calm and graceful. Yoga improves posture dramatically and enhances natural movement without which no woman, no matter how fit, can be elegant.

Kari-Ann Moller has been practising yoga for twelve years and its importance is such that she squeezes an extra hour out of the day to make sure she has time for a daily workout. *"I get up an hour before the children do,"* she says. *"That's pretty early but I must do my exercises and breathing undisturbed and peacefully. Yoga awakens me in my own time. My mind and body comes to life gradually and I always feel very strong and energised after a workout, but relaxed at the same time. Yoga leaves you full of energy and alert, but also full of inner tranquillity. It's the best preparation for whatever demands and stresses the day might bring."*

Pat Knight has just discovered yoga and has fallen for its physical and mental benefits. *"It generates inner serenity and confidence and, consequently, self-respect,"* she says with the enthusiasm of the newly converted.

There are other toning and relaxation techniques – and the relaxation aspect of exercise is highly beneficial to older women – available besides yoga, depending on the number of

Exercise

qualified practitioners within your reach, geographically and financially.

These include **Pilates**, in which muscles are worked individually in harmony with breathing exercises; the **Alexander Technique**, which works on correctly aligning the spine and body carriage to lessen ageing and damaging tension and stress; and **Medau**, a relative newcomer to the public's attention, a combination of aerobics, breathing and stretching exercises. All are good for older women because they emphasise developing strength and flexibility as opposed to skill and speed.

Some exercise is pure pleasure, dancing for one. A fifty-year-old who took it up, going to a local club twice a week for a night of whirling around the floor, said she'd forgotten *"how jolly moving about feels. It raises your spirits and really is quite a workout. I've felt more energetic about everything since."* "Moving about" has a youthful vigour that sitting watching television lacks. Dancing energetically can use up seven calories a minute, if you're counting, compared with mopping the floor – three calories a minute – so put down the mop, shrug off your sluggishness and take to the dance floor.

It doesn't have to be "Come Dancing" at the club if that's not your style. Kari-Ann Moller discovered "earth dancing" last year, an American import which is sure to catch on with women of all ages. *"It brings your spirit into a lot of free form movement,"* she explains. *"There's no rigidity, no rules, so it's very relaxing and liberating; you flow with your own rhythm. When I went to the first session there were babies and grandmothers joining in so there's no age restriction and no ability level to start. Wonderful for women who are just warming up to the idea of movement and exercise. My children roll their eyes a bit when I talk about it, but they're so conservative. At my age I don't have to be conservative. This kind of dancing makes you feel very empowered and in control, very strong and free, all good things for women at a turning point or time of change in their lives. Feeling free is very like feeling young."*

Whatever kind of exercise you choose – and it's vital to do something to sustain the elements of youth in your body, not hasten the bending to time – it should be something that not only has personal appeal, but is practically possible. There's no point signing up for swimming time if the baths are miles from you and you have to change buses to get there. The first bit of foul weather or feeling tired will scupper your good intentions. Likewise, an expensive course of fancy exercises will become an additional pressure to keep up rather than a pleasure to enjoy if it's straining the budget to pay for them. Exercise will become, if it's not already, a natural part of daily life so give it some thought before setting out. The energy it generates spills out into other areas of life, making you a more active friend, energetic lover, interested parent, an all-round more relaxed, confident and healthy being. Working your body means your body will work for you.

Are you physically elegant?
◆ You are if you can bend, stretch, twist and reach smoothly, easily and fluidly; if you can glide rather than step awkwardly into a room; if you gracefully skirt a gasping jogger on the path with leg cramp without breaking your stride.
◆ You are not elegant if you play the show-off and stride past a panting runner twenty years younger than yourself; if you creak in bed; if you can't bend comfortably to give yourself a pedicure.

3 ◆ *General Health*

"Look to your health; and if you have it . . . value it . . . for health is the . . . blessing that money cannot buy."

When Izaak Walton wrote those words more than three hundred years ago, good health was mostly a matter of luck. You were lucky not to be caught in a war or a plague-ridden city; lucky not to be beaten by your master or die in childbirth; lucky to survive having a tooth pulled, measles or an accusation of witchcraft. About the only way to guarantee good health was not to get sick and stay out of the way – maybe that's why Walton went fishing so often.

These days good health is a matter of valuing and looking after your whole self, physical, emotional and mental. Inner health is not divorced from outer, as the good health of one feeds the other.

Many doctors and gerontologists agree that in the past there has been too much emphasis on chronological ageing. Good health depends not so much on how many calendar years your body's been around, but what it's done and what's been done to it. If you've stuffed it full of fat, tobacco, beer and tranquillisers for years, it's likely to protest a bit now. If it's been reasonably well treated and respected, it's capable of continuing enthusiastically on. The human body is astonishing in its resilience; even years of punishment won't rob it entirely of its vitality and survival instincts, and it's never too late to begin taking better care of it.

Your real enemy is a cowardly and defeatist attitude which equates ageing with withering away. This is dangerous rubbish in these modern scientific times which offer much to support body and spirit; but the first step to a pleasurable and energetic later life is a concerted effort to maintain good health. It has nothing to do with vanity and everything to do with survival. Healthy people live longer and better; the unfit and unwell, who are also the unhappy, live more uncomfortably, die earlier.

Your body's true age is determined by diet, exercise, its ability to fight off infection and cope with stress, its emotional and social outlets and protection from ageing environmental factors like exposure to sun and pollution. Although a woman will go out and spend the grocery money on a new anti-ageing cream, she'll overlook or ignore the routine preventative medicine readily available from her own doctor. Unlike women in some other countries, notably North America, women in the UK show great resistance to going regularly to a doctor for a "good health" or "well woman" check-up. Doctors, they insist, are for times when you're ill, exhibiting symptoms.

A woman feeling the need to pull a new image together wouldn't hesitate to have her outward self fine-tuned at the beauty salon: new hairstyle, facial, pedicure and manicure, wax, make-up, but she'd think twice about checking the equipment under the skin. One of the best and most valuable presents a woman can treat herself to is a complete physical check-up, either through a well woman clinic, if such a service is available, or privately, if she can afford it. It's unlikely to cost more than the car's annual MOT overhaul, but will give her lasting confidence and peace of mind about her own health and possibly uncover incipient problems. "Feeling fine" is no reason to reject a thorough investigation of your health. Some of the age-related illnesses have invisible symptoms.

The first inkling of hypertension, or high blood pressure, for example, may be when it fells you with a stroke. A regular thorough check-up will give you and your doctor a fair reading of your general health and pick out any potential problems. It's also an opportunity to discuss any new symptoms or feelings about growing older that are troubling you, and be reassured. Some tests for specific conditions are advisable as you get older. Women should know what they

General Health

are and why they're necessary, not to frighten themselves but to ensure they catch and halt serious complaints in the early, curable stages. You should know what tests are recommended so you can talk knowledgeably to your GP and feel the two of you are a team working for your better health. Most doctors these days welcome and are sympathetic to discussing the fears and concerns of middle-aged patients and won't dismiss your worries lightly.

If you're unlucky enough to have a doctor who is reluctant to actively pursue preventative health, or not interested in discussing your health with you, seriously consider changing to a more open-minded and up-to-date practitioner. Doctors are not immune from the social prejudice that sees ageing as inevitable and unchangeable no matter what age it starts, and urge acceptance rather than resistance to unnecessary slowing down. A doctor who's more interested in keeping patients fit and fighting rather than accepting time's changes is more your style. Every doctor should be keen to offer most of the following, or suggest patients at least consider them:

Blood pressure test: From middle-age onwards, it is advisable to have your blood pressure tested as hypertension is undetectable without a test. There are no outward symptoms and outward temperament is not a reliable guide. The red-faced, loud-voiced committee chairwoman may have normal blood pressure while the mild-mannered librarian who scarcely raises her voice at all may need medication to control hers. An average pressure reading is 120/80. Some people actually have low blood pressure, usually considered a medical benefit, but anything higher than the average will be monitored. If yours does register in the danger zone, your GP may decide to first try and regulate it through diet with a low-fat, low-salt regime. Failing that, the most common treatment is prescription drugs. Some experimentation may be necessary to find the right kind and dosage of tablets, but this is common. Side effects such as changes in sleep patterns, leg cramps or fluid retention are also possible but you don't have to meekly accept them. Discuss any side effects with your doctor who may be able to alter the tablets to ones more suitable to you.

Electrocardiogram (ECG): This provides a read-out of the heart's pumping action and shows up abnormalities. A blood test is often done at the same time to check for raised levels of cholesterol, an indication of potential heart disease and also blood glucose and triglyceride levels as well as a general screen for any blood abnormalities. As the point of preventative medicine is to warn you of trouble in advance, this may be the most valuable test you have.

Although women complain that these tests are "stressful", it really is too late in life to cling to such a childish, head-in-the-sand attitude. Knowledge is power in health, as in other areas of life, and knowing exactly what shape you're in gives you the opportunity to head off danger and repair damage.

Cervical smear: The last few years have seen an intensive campaign by doctors and health authorities to encourage women to have this simple, painless test, which involves scraping a few cells off the cervix and sending them to a lab for signs of abnormality. Why then do women resist it so? Part of the fault lies with the medical spokesmen who introduced it as a "cancer test" – nobody wants to be tested and told they have cancer. It is not a cancer test: it is a test for several abnormalities, one of which may be cervical cancer, or its precancerous cell changes. If caught in the early stages, cervical cancer is curable, hence the pressure on women for early detection.

Labelling it a "smear" test didn't make it any more attractive either, conjuring up all sorts of messy, inelegant images. Embarrassment, false modesty and fear hold enough women back without an image problem too. It's a shame some women feel so squeamish or sensitive about it, but it doesn't make the test any less necessary. Most doctors recommend that women over forty continue to be tested every three to five years, although doctors discontinue testing in a patient's mid-sixties if all previous tests have been negative. Part of this examination should be a manual pelvic inspection, in which the doctor feels for benign growths called fibroids, and cysts. Even more thorough is an ultrasound scan, similar to that used on pregnant women, which will show up abnormalities. It does not involve radiation and may be available at hospital clinics

General Health

on the NHS. Failing that, some women may feel it's worth having this done privately. If the thought of this really upsets you, you can minimise the awkwardness factor by choosing a woman GP or going to a well woman clinic where they tend to be more sensitive and understanding of any discomfort and embarrassment a woman may feel. It's tough for any woman, even the most authoritative company president, to be in full command of herself and circumstances and to feel at an advantage with her feet in the stirrups.

Mammogram: *"Like pâté under glass"* is how one woman described her experience of a mammogram and seeing her breast squashed between two glass plates. A mammogram is a special X-ray of breast tissue that shows up lumps undetectable by touch. Don't be put off by stories from women who emphasise the pain of the experience. It *is* uncomfortable, but the discomfort is momentary and far outweighed by the possible breast – and/or life-saving benefits of early detection. In addition to a mammogram women should continue to examine their own breasts every month even after they reach menopause. It takes minutes and could add years to your life, if you find a cancerous lump early. Women who until now have not made a habit of regularly examining themselves may look at their reflection in the mirror and conclude something's amiss. The mental image of perfect, rounded breasts is more image than reality.

Most breasts are irregular: one may be larger than the other or noticeably higher. Under inexperienced fingers they may feel too "lumpy" but a healthy breast can feel as lumpy as an old camp-bed mattress. Until you've been examining your breasts for some months you won't be able to tell what's normal in shape and feel for you and will be unaware of small irregularities. To physically examine your own breasts, press firmly around each, above and beneath, with the flat part of the fingers. Booklets on breast self-examination are available from any GP's office. Better yet, get the practice nurse to show you how. If you feel a lump in the tissue that doesn't budge, consult your doctor. Dimpled or puckered skin around the nipple, discharge from the nipple or swelling of the lymph glands which run from the breast to the armpit, are also signals a doctor should be seen. Even if there is a lump that requires medical attention, don't get the weepies; the majority of lumps removed for a biopsy (laboratory testing of the tissue) are harmless. Harmless or not, better out than in.

Glaucoma test: Glaucoma is another of the symptomless troubles that plague the mature years. No obvious symptoms other than, in some cases, a halo around bright objects, no pain, and suddenly, no proper vision. Between the ages of forty and fifty all women should be tested for glaucoma which if left untreated can lead to loss of peripheral vision and "tunnel" vision. If the disease runs in your family you should have had your eyes tested in your thirties – so if this is news to you, visit an ophthalmic optician as soon as possible. Glaucoma is the result of the fluid balance in the eye altering and putting pressure on the eyeball. Eventually it presses on the optic nerve and narrows the field of vision. Prescription drugs and occasionally surgery to relieve the pressure can control it.

Cataracts: After forty, most opticians will check automatically for signs of cataracts, although most sufferers are in their sixties and seventies. Cataracts cloud or mist the focusing lens of the eye, creating blurred vision. Surgery can correct it.

Sight test: A sure sign of reaching middle life is having to hold the newspaper a foot away to read it. Everyone requires a sight test some time between the ages of forty and fifty as their ability to focus at close range diminishes. No matter how perfect your vision has been in the past, you will require reading glasses in your future. It has nothing to do with being long- or short-sighted, as it is a natural change in the eye that happens with age regardless of how good or poor your vision has been. Reading glasses may be a nuisance to adjust to for the woman who's never worn spectacles, but for regular wearers of glasses the constant switching between those for seeing distance and those for reading menus and price tags prompts many a woman to consider contact lenses for her distance viewing. All contact lenses must be fitted by a qualified optician and all require rigorous care to keep them clean and free from infection-causing bacteria. To the uninitiated, the cleaning, soaking and general care systems sound daunting but in no time it becomes as routine and un-

General Health

remarkable as cleaning your teeth. One tip from Frances Meachem, which will be echoed by any lens wearer who's spent a frantic quarter-hour with her nose in the sink or crawling over the bathroom lino searching for a lost lens: get them tinted. It doesn't affect everyday vision and when they do fall into the sink or on to the counter, you can easily spot them.

Novices should be warned that while contact lenses are valued as one of the marvels of the modern age by women liberated from specs, occasionally bits of dirt or grit or mascara get into the eye, under the lens, and cause needle stabs of pain. Lens wearers tend to wink frantically if they feel a bit of stray grit in their eye, in order to dislodge it before it gets near the lens. Total strangers in trains, restaurants and check-out queues become convinced you're winking at them – life becomes very interesting when you give up glasses for lenses.

There are several types of lenses, and the ones you want are the ones most comfortable for you to wear, professionally fitted. Many women will have tried lenses years ago, in the era of the hard lens; things have changed for the better:

◆ Corneal lenses are gas permeable, which means oxygen gets through to the eye-making them easier to tolerate than the old hard lens;
◆ Hydrophilic or soft lenses need more care than gas permeable ones and have to be replaced more often, but wearers claim the comfort factor is worth it;
◆ Extended wear lenses can be left in overnight (all others must be removed before sleep) but need to be scrupulously monitored. The jury's still out on them and some ophthalmologists are reluctant to recommend them;
◆ Disposable lenses are now readily available but also need scrupulous monitoring and many ophthalmologists feel more research is needed.

But by all means, ask everywhere, get all the information and opinion you can, and make your own decision.

Menopause: All these tests may tell you you're in great shape, good health and ready to face the future with optimism and energy. But every woman, no matter what the state of her general health, faces her own crisis in mid-life: the menopause is a watershed beside which other health considerations pale for many women. Although many women express relief at being past child-bearing age, most women experience feelings of loss at this dramatic change in themselves. Menopause generally happens between the ages of forty-five and fifty-five. Women approaching it or in the midst of it find their premenstrual symptoms occur with a vengeance: depression, fatigue, irritability and general unwellness. They may suffer the familiar hot flushes, night sweats and mood swings. The dropping oestrogen levels in the body leave vaginal tissues drier and thinner, so sex may be uncomfortable, affecting not only the woman, but her partner.

Those who suffer needn't accept their fate. Never "not bother" to consult your GP because what you're going through is "natural". Childbirth is natural but few women go through it without some form of analgesic. *Dying* is natural, but we tend to fight it off as long as possible.

The menopause is as much a psychological turning point as a physical one. It's a blow for a woman to reach the end of her reproductive life, whether or not she wants more children, or even has any children. Fecundity is intensely bound up with women's sexuality and the menopause robs her of the choice or option to ever have any more children. Fear of waning sexual interest, her own or her partner's, also haunts women at this time. Nature is cruel, but mankind is cunning and today there is no reason for any woman to suffer when medical help is readily available. Unless there are medical restrictions, such as a previous history of blood clots or breast cancer, a doctor will usually recommend a course of Hormone Replacement Therapy, or HRT. Whether taken as a tablet, injection or implant, HRT is generally a combination of the hormones oestrogen and progesterone. Earlier hormone therapies which contained just oestrogen posed the risk of womb cancer, but the addition of progesterone protects against it. Women converted to the benefits of HRT refer to it as a miracle cure. Menopausal symptoms vanish overnight, the depression and general debility lifts and sexual symptoms abate. *"Taking* HRT *is like returning from the dead,"* says one convert. HRT also combats osteoporosis, the bone thinning

General Health

disease that leads to brittle bones and the hunched, humped posture of the "elderly". Doctors can now measure bone mineral density with radiation dosages of less than one tenth of a chest X-ray, giving them information about the bones before and after menopause. It also protects against heart disease, leading some scientists to credit it with being a true anti-ageing formula. Women considering HRT should know that it will cause monthly bleeding to return and that some women experience strong adolescent-style cramps with it, but all this should be discussed with your doctor or gynaecologist. If you're met with a blank refusal to constructive help, you could consider switching to a more sympathetic and aware practitioner. Menopausal treatment is a highly specialised field and help, in some form, is available.

If your medical history makes taking HRT impossible, there are other remedies to relieve menopausal distress. Help your body through its hormonal turmoil by cutting out caffeine and alcohol, heavily sugared and spiced foods, all things that trigger body temperature changes and affect moods. Throw out the synthetic underwear and sheets and switch to pure cotton which will absorb perspiration more easily and feel cooler. The antidote to vaginal dryness is a welcome one: regular sex, but if it's too uncomfortable, KY jelly or equivalent, an old friend from the uncomfortable post-natal days, makes a reappearance in the bathroom cabinet. If all else fails, consult a homeopath. Many women find great relief in homeopathic remedies and most are pleasant to use. Some of it may be psychological: one woman said she preferred combating nature with nature, but whatever soothes the symptoms is right.

Insomnia: One unlooked-for difficulty as you get older is insomnia, or an inability to sleep. Sleep may become increasingly difficult to relax into although women complain of feeling tired and catnap in the afternoon. *"I think,"* jokes an active sixty-five-year-old, *"you don't sleep at night so well because your body's afraid if it goes to sleep it will forget to wake up!"*

Although many women would agree with Sandra Paul's lament that *"you never seem to get enough sleep"*, the actual number of hours needed differs from body to body. The eight-hours-a-night rule can't apply to the executive traveller, politician, new mother, or university reveller, all of whom manage for days, even weeks, on three or four hours. Others can barely function without a full nine or ten hours.

Anyone who has suffered a bout of insomnia will recognise sleep is as essential for good health as diet and medical care. Sleep nourishes the body just as food does. While bodies sleep the maintenance crews come out, repairing the ravages of the day by mending cells, boosting immunity and levelling out stress.

Body rhythms fluctuate as regularly as sea tides and sleep is an important part of the pattern. The heart rate slows down, as does blood pressure and breathing, and the body temperature drops. Digestion slows. In sleep the body recoups its resources and marshals its strength for the next day's wear and tear. Sleeplessness shows clearly in dull skin, dark-circled eyes, depressed posture and general irritability. No matter how skilfully you do your make-up, lack of sleep shows in a general flatness. And yes, it is ageing: even young faces sag from prolonged tiredness.

In times of stress or a crisis, sleep is a great soother and it's this quality of comfort, repose and refreshment that is sought after by the sleepless. Nothing is so frustrating and wearying as lying in the darkness longing for sleep but unable to shut out the events of the day. Women often find in the years of change and reassessment that sleep is no longer the easy, natural, unforced thing it was. *"My greatest difficulties sleeping were during the years of trying to be Supermum,"* recalls Frances Meachem. *"I had too much to do; the house, the family, my work. I felt, like a lot of women, that everything had to be perfect. I felt I ought to get up at four a.m. to make the tea. I did resort to sleeping pills at one point but hated it. Then I found that if I got up instead of lying there fretting and made a list of all the things I had to do, it calmed me. My mind would relax once I'd drawn up a game plan and knew how I was going to attack the next day."*

Many older women find sleep elusive because they're not really tired enough, says Kari-Ann Moller. If growing older

General Health

means giving up some physical activities, the body has surplus energy that needs to be let go of before bedtime. *"Feeling weary from inactivity or boredom is very debilitating,"* she says. *"Gentle exercise like walking or yoga takes away that low feeling and lets the body unwind naturally before sleep."*

Real insomnia is a serious problem that knocks the stuffing out of life. Endless hours pacing the floor, or staring out at the dark street and quiet houses, or lying open-eyed and tense on the bed is no preparation for a good day ahead. Pills and tranquillisers are not an answer, except perhaps in the short term after a shock or crisis, but another problem. Insomnia can be attacked methodically, starting with a firm pep talk to yourself about putting the day's troubles aside when you enter the bedroom. Your nights are only as good as your days, and if you load up with problems, responsibilities and a lot of unnecessary emotional clutter you will be unable to clear your mind for sleep. Find a relaxing and different activity for the evening: if your day involves sedentary pursuits and a lot of reading, go for a walk, swim or game of bowls. If you've had a physically demanding day, read, listen to music or have a soothing bath. If you've been house-bound for days, have a night out – anything that breaks the lethargic pattern lightens the spirit and makes sleep more possible. A drink before bed should be non-alcoholic and non-caffeinated. Whisky, coffee and tea are stimulants. Don't eat spicy or hard-to-digest foods because no matter how tired the rest of you is, your stomach will probably stay up to complain.

You might do an inventory of your sleeping arrangements: has your mattress gone lumpy and you hadn't noticed? Would one more or one less pillow make any difference? Are you away from distracting background noise? Is the room too hot, too cool, too airless. Has your partner become noisier? This is one of the great difficulties of growing older together, that if one is restless, the other tends to suffer too. Women remark that their once silent bed-mates suddenly start annoying new habits of snoring, breathing heavily or grinding their teeth, and are generally more restless than they were when they were younger.

Making your sleeping quarters as attractive and enticing as

possible helps. Crisp, clean sheets, a pretty, airy room, a feeling of peace engendered by *not* having a pile of guilt-producing ironing stacked in a corner, and the warmth and comfort of the (quiet) person beside you, should lure you into letting down your defences and sinking into sleep.

Stress: Good health is not just about smooth physical functioning. Emotional and mental health are as vital, and that means learning to manage stress. Stress is a great robber of sleep, as it is a great robber of most of the pleasures in life. The only person who doesn't suffer from stress is a dead person, so learning to recognise good and bad stress and cope with both is a life skill. If a situation makes you edgy, worried, even panicky, it's labelled bad stress. If you feel on your mettle, apprehensive but not anxious, and equal to it, it's good stress and called a challenge. One woman's stress is another woman's challenge, and the difference is largely one of attitude. Unless you see stressful situations as challenges to conquer, the pressure can wear you down and out. It will furrow your brow, turn down the corners of your mouth, and manifest itself in overeating, sleeplessness, lower resistance to illness, hair loss or loss of libido.

Personality types come into play with stress. Some women are grand at handling big, life-affecting situations, sudden disasters and emergencies, but go mad over the daily trivia and aggravations that scarcely ruffle another woman. Some women are unfazed at everyday setbacks, hold-ups and let-downs and fall apart when confronted with a major issue. Much of how we react depends on how in control of the situation we feel. No matter how potentially stressful – a wedding, a new job, a first date – we feel excited and optimistic if we feel we can handle it and control it to some degree. If something feels beyond us, despair and fear sets in, control slips through our fingers and we feel all the stress of the situation.

Seeing grown children leaving the family home for university, a job or marriage is stressful; some women might see this as a loss and feel neglected and fearful of the future without their children. Another woman in the same situation might see it as the beginning of new freedom for herself and

General Health

new life for her self-reliant children. The stress is not so much in the situation but in our reaction to it.

Most women in these middle years face some major stresses: a spouse may be retiring or being made redundant; she herself may be contemplating an upheaval in her own circumstances, a return to work or education; a divorce, or the death of an elderly parent, or even her spouse, may come unexpectedly. Nearly all women experience some unease at what they fear is their loss of physical attractiveness as they grow older. If a woman has always been attractive, and used to admiration, it may be even harder.

Whatever fears sadden and worry them, women often find it difficult to talk about their stresses or to get much support or sympathy if they do voice them at home. In most households, the woman is the emotional linchpin – everyone else brings their emotional crises and stresses to her, while she nurses hers in private. As the comforter and shorer-up of sagging egos, she's hardly recognised as having real stresses of her own, often until she is at the breaking point. One woman, looking back over her family life, could see how much everyone leaned on her and how impossible it was to voice the pressures she felt. *"My husband assumed I'd support him in all his emotional upheavals with his job, which I did, and the children needed support and encouragement which I gave willingly, and my own mother was devastated when my father left her and needed a shoulder to cry on – and sometimes my Dad did too because he felt guilty – sometimes I used to sit in the bath and cry, but I couldn't tell anybody how overburdened and weighted down I felt. Everyone got better as time passed and the children got older of course . . . but even today nobody asks how I feel, how I cope."*

A woman's best source of emotional support may be her friends, whose stress-deflating kindnesses, sympathy and shared experiences bolster many a woman who feels she's taken on (or is giving) too much.

Stress, like any other problem, has its solutions: walking away from it, or burying it, aren't solutions at all. Learning to cope with it is. If you feel constantly under the gun and overpressured it's worth taking stock of how you got into this situation and start making plans to get out. Being in control is elegant; desperation isn't.

Stress-inducing situations and how to cope with them:
◆ Are there too many changes in your life all at once? Moving house, a new job, a divorce, leaving a job, a health crisis – one of them at a time is enough for any woman. Don't change jobs, move house, take a new lover or decide to have a late baby at forty-five all in the same week.
◆ Do you have a perspective on life? Is it always a major crisis, no matter what the incident – when a pot boils over, when you miss a bus, when a child fails his exams, when your husband suggests separate vacations this year? Some things are crises – others shouldn't bite so deep. If you fall apart over every upset you really will wear out your heart valves. It's time to step back and reassess your view of things so you can see the difference between things that can be fixed in five minutes with a damp cloth and things that will leave a scar for years. Some things were made to go berserk over and others to shrug off. Whether you shrug off the boiled pot or the departed husband is up to you.
◆ Can you establish priorities? In major corporations they run seminars for senior executives on time management. It's a way of establishing control and priorities. Another way to manage, as all senior executives are told, is to make a list. Lists force you to set priorities and control time. Saying there's not enough time is meaningless. Everyone has exactly the same amount of time: twenty-four hours a day. Organisation imposes control. Head your list with the things that absolutely have to get done, followed in descending order by the things that should be done, would be nice if they got done, and won't kill anyone if they don't get done. Seeing it in black and white clarifies a situation wonderfully. Not all stressful issues can of course be solved like this – some, like a difficult relationship with a spouse or child, or health or financial worries, don't clear away on a list, but you can map out how much time you'll

General Health

spend worrying about it or discussing it that day, or set aside time to confront the person about it, or simply think about it, uninterrupted by other issues for an hour.

◆ Can you give yourself a respite, however brief? After you've done everything you can in a crisis – had a cry, done all the practical things, talked to everyone who needed to be talked to – it's time to tune out and focus on something else, preferably pleasurable, even for a brief time. Parents of ill children or mourners at a funeral sometimes erupt into levity and apparent frivolousness and are criticised for it. Nothing could be more unjust. This kind of breaking out is self-defence of the most basic kind, a safeguard against mental and emotional breakdown, a release from the terrible stress of the moment. In less extreme, but still stressful circumstances, you can afford to mentally shut out the world and steal some time for yourself, to be at peace over a book, in the garden, on a long walk.

◆ Do you give yourself time alone? It's the number one de-stresser on many a stressed-out woman's list. If you're rich, run to a spa; if you're not, lock yourself in the bathroom, fill the tub, soak and dream. Every woman needs time to reflect and be offstage and inaccessible to the world, however briefly. It's worth cultivating in private moments a long-term view of life and your philosophy about present troubles – whatever the crisis, what will it all matter a hundred years from now?

Depression: One of the common side effects of stress is depression. Serious depression may require professional counselling but most women can pull themselves out of it by activity and reaching out for others. It's not easy to stay depressed when your body's working hard, which is why exercise is such a brilliant cure for depression. So is spring cleaning, whatever the season. Turning out all the cupboards, all the wardrobes, attacking the garden and savagely pulling out all those weeds is cathartic. Physically it exercises and tires you; mentally you're imposing order on chaos which is very satisfying; emotionally you're accomplishing something which is gratifying. Good friends are the other best prescription for depression. They repair self-esteem and offer hope and listen to you uncritically.

Occasionally depression gets such a grip that all the well-meaning friends and self-exorcism have no effect. The time for professional counselling has arrived. Your doctor is usually the first one to see in seeking help. Many general practices now have a resident counsellor or an association with psychotherapy groups, either individual practices or groups connected with a local hospital, and a GP can recommend or set up an appointment to see a counsellor or therapist. Just the sound of a therapist frightens some women off, but any stigma attached to mental or emotional breakdowns or fragility is rapidly lifting. Everyone feels overwhelmed by the burdens and pressures of life and if the pressure hits at a particularly weak moment in your life, there's no shame in seeking help to bolster your defences. At one time it was fashionable to fob off depressed women with tranquillisers; today's treatment is more likely to be a sympathetic and encouraging discussion to root out the source of the depression, rather than suppress it with drugs. Depression is often caused by feelings about the world at large, and your own world in particular is overbalanced on the downside; counselling rights the balance and restores perspective. It helps a woman see and accept that there is also goodness and rightness and positiveness in her life.

Women are prey, as they get older, to the phenomenon of social ageing. Too often older people find themselves cut off by circumstances (the death of a spouse, divorce, a move, far-flung family) from mixing with other people. Humans need other humans. Without that contact, older women may grow isolated, out of touch and lonely, all of which is prematurely ageing. Worst of all it may not be recognised as loneliness – family, even a family doctor, may dismiss the woman's slightly wandering thoughts or disinclination to go out as natural signs of age. There's nothing natural about being cut off from other people. The telly is no substitute for live, argumentative, interesting, gossipy people. Like any other human faculty, if you don't use the brain – in conversation, in learning new things, in experiencing new situations – it starts

General Health

to slow down and fall into disuse. Being with other people is stimulating, builds confidence and is rejuvenating, and sociability is a big part of general good health.

Alternative Medicine: Most women depend on modern science and medicine for their physical well-being but sometimes the medical establishment hasn't the answers they seek. A growing number turn to alternative medicine, and far from being a sort of medical lunatic fringe, some doctors now include homeopathic remedies in their general practice. Homeopathic medicine is based on the premise of treating the whole person, not just the symptoms, so most homeopathic practitioners will question you closely about the general state of your health before prescribing anything. Some women swear by their gentle and effective remedies which are mixtures and different strengths of naturally occurring minerals and salts; the emotional power of believing in your medicine is healing in itself. If you don't want a detailed consultation with an actual practitioner, chemists, health food shops and supermarkets carry some homeopathic remedies.

Offshoots of the search for natural healing, for both body and soul, include Bach flower remedies, and aromatherapy, in which essential plant oils are massaged into the skin to relieve symptoms – rosemary around the temples for stress and tiredness, for example; reflexology, in which a practitioner examines the soles of the feet to find pressure points corresponding to body organs which are then massaged and made better; iridology, at the other end of the body, in which the iris and its markings in the eye can be read like a map of body areas and upsets and weaknesses pinpointed; and acupuncture, for which you *must* see a qualified acupuncturist, who will treat illness by pushing special needles into parts of a patient's body which are claimed to cause changes in the flow of chemicals and energy and promote healing. Acupuncture is said to be effective in overcoming behavioural problems such as smoking or overeating, or continuing difficulties such as chronic indigestion and constipation.

The best medicine for good general health is to be happy – which sounds so much easier than it is for many women in real life. You can't force yourself to be happy and you can't force the people or the circumstances that make you unhappy to change, but you can cut down on the pressures that sap much of the joy from life. Women are notoriously bad at saying no to anyone, but it's time to start if you want to have any time and life to yourself.

You needn't take on all the responsibility for everyone else's happiness. They'll have to find their own, for themselves, without you. This is particularly difficult for women who have been at the family centre for years, but it's time you took your happiness as seriously as you've always taken theirs. As you reach this middle stage in life, some reassessment is in order, and some clarification of your own identity:

Do you really know yourself and like yourself; do the people closest to you see you as a person, or a title – *you*, or just Mother or Wife? Do they respect the things that are important to you, give you time to indulge them, encourage you to do more? Are they emotionally expressive, so affection isn't a one-way street from you to them? Have you come to terms with your own regrets and mistakes of the past? Now is the time to reorder your life, for your own good health, and to be kind and just to yourself. Looking back, you must be able to see, in order to be happy, that you did the best you could with what you had at the time. No one could do better. And now you can look forward.

◆ **Most Inelegant Medical Crime:** Smoking, without a doubt. It suffocates the lungs, yellows your teeth, poisons your breath and creates a cloud of unwanted perfume around you: Ashtray No. 1.

◆ **Most Elegant Mantra to chant under stress:** *"Never sweat the small stuff . . . it's all small stuff."*

4 ♦ *Sex*

Sex assumes an importance out of all perspective when women reach the watershed of mid-life, rather the way it does in adolescence when sexual fervour overrides relationships with parents, friends, school work and hobbies. After the first, furious flurry of adolescent discovery, sex becomes part of normal life in your twenties and thirties; a decade or two later, you're reassessing its role again, and it becomes An Issue. Like the teenage years, mid-life is a time of sexual upheaval and change, although this time the hormones are all on the other side of the street, retreating rather than surging forward. Many women assume that whatever other benefits the years bring – stability, self-knowledge, assurance – they won't be sexual. It comes as a pleasant discovery that interest can be as high as ever and performance, if anything, better.

Youth does not have a monopoly on sex although you would have a difficult time persuading advertisers of that. As long as you're still breathing you're a sexual being and, like food and exercise, sex is part of a healthy lifestyle. You never outgrow the need for physical contact and emotional fulfilment and the thrill of arousing someone who also arouses you. Frances Meachem recalls a story she once read in a newspaper about a seventy-eight-year-old man who stabbed his wife of the same age because he thought she was being unfaithful. "It gives us all hope," she says.

It's not impossible to live without sex – the libido, like anything else, fades and weakens without regular use, but sex is important not for the physical act itself, but because of the intimacy, acceptance and affirmation of our desirability that goes with it.

The difficulties of the menopause, dealt with in the previous chapter, force sex to Issue status; once they're accepted and dealt with, a woman's sex life is as rich as it ever was and is as fulfilling as she chooses to make it. At this age, says Pat Knight, a woman's sexuality is *"more of a slow burn than a roaring fire but the need to get and give warmth is there."*

Older women have a sexual magic their younger sisters lack. To men they are more of a sexual mystery than younger women. They've had time to have many experiences with men, not just sexual, which makes them intriguing. Younger women may try and counteract this by doing things more energetically but they don't necessarily do them better. Where young women may have more frenetic sexual energy, older women have gained a more deeply satisfying sensuality. Being an assured, accomplished and experienced woman, you no longer need to prove anything in bed.

At this age, you know your sexual preferences (although sex is a bit like food: there's always something you haven't tried) and no longer worry about being compared and judged between the sheets. *"A lot of my single life in my twenties seemed to be spent comparing sexual notes with girlfriends and I always felt my card was marked 'could do better',"* recalls a forty-five-year-old. *"Everybody seemed to be part of a big contest to be best in bed. There was a lot of pressure to be free and liberated and always brilliant in bed. My first thought after making love was 'I wonder if the last girl he slept with was better than me'. It's laughable now, but I worried about sex more than I enjoyed it."*

Sex in the second inning of life is definitely more relaxed – *"The pressure is off to perform,"* as Frances Meachem says – although it doesn't lose its importance. Many women find their enthusiasm for sex returns after years of indifference or lack of opportunities. As one woman expressed it, *"I wasn't negative about sex in my thirties and early forties, I was neutral. There was so much else going on, everything was so hectic, I didn't have time for it. I had a demanding job, two children and a house to run; the pressure was incredible and time was eaten up. I was exhausted from work and the*

Sex

children's demands and wanted to black out at night. I forgot about sex. It was a wonderful rediscovery though. I work part-time now, the children have left home, and my husband's not as caught up in his career either. It's like finding a favourite toy after years of it being buried away in the attic!"

Why then do some women turn off or turn away from sex as though reaching "a certain age" cut off the need for physical affirmation of a relationship and their own attractiveness and physical power? Insecurity, either about performance or physical appearance, is usually the culprit. Despite the sexual revolution and an avalanche of information about sex in books, magazines, and manuals with as much illustrated detail and step-by-step instruction as other DIY manuals, basically you're alone in the bedroom and left to sort out what you need, have read about, feel, would like with a partner you don't want to frighten and do want to please. It's one of the enduring myths both sexes labour under that everyone else is doing it more, doing it better and enjoying it more than you and your partner. The only time we witness sexual engagement is on film, and that often compounds insecurity. Onscreen lovers are invariably young, taut, smooth-skinned, with flat stomachs and perfect breasts and bottoms. They are filmed in flattering light from arousing angles.

You know this is complete fiction because (a) their make-up doesn't smudge and (b) the earth *always* moves, but it doesn't make you feel confident about revealing your fifty-year-old body when your partner has been watching a twenty-year-old thrashing about in seamless perfection. Comparisons make everybody cringe.

Sexual confidence at any age starts with liking your physical self. If your primary concern is to hide and cover up, it's going to inhibit sexual activity no end. For years you may have walked naked across the bedroom in perfect comfort, pride even, then suddenly you catch sight of crepey thighs in the mirror or are struck by how gravity has seized your bottom; it seems kinder to everyone to slip on a nightie. If at twenty you welcomed mirrors on the ceiling, you'll long for decorative plasterwork now. And sex in the dark is suddenly more appealing than at high noon with every enlarged pore and wrinkle exposed to merciless sunlight.

"The ageing process is much harder on women than men," Sandra Paul admits. "An elegant woman has to work harder to keep her allure because there is still a double standard. Men are seen to be attractive as they age but women are often seen to be merely older although that is changing because there are so many wonderful-looking older women around now.

"But I do think women go off sex if they are dissatisfied with their appearance. If you're a bit overweight or wrinkly you're made so conscious of it by the smooth, impossible bodies in magazines or even memories of yourself at twenty. You can't change everything about the way you look but you can change your attitude."

Changing how you feel about your body may be more important than losing a few pounds or doing waist-bends to tighten your midriff. Bodies that show their age show only they've been lived in and loved. And if that body is strong and supple and capable of giving and receiving pleasure, it's a cause for pride not shame. "*My wrinkles and lines are maps of pleasure,*" says an older woman with panache.

There are, sadly, still women who feel sex is something that belongs to a youthful past and that the menopause is nature's way of telling a woman her time is up. More than one woman has described an active sex life as *"inappropriate"* at her time of life. *"We're past all that now,"* must be one of the saddest and bitterest comments on a relationship and a totally false one: no one is "past" needing human touch, physical expression and intimacy. It's true you may have to give up swinging from the chandelier for less strenuous sexual games but nobody outgrows the need to be held and desired. *"Feeling desirable, sexy and being wanted keeps up morale and confidence,"* Frances Meachem says. *"Being loved is rejuvenating."*

Women who share an active relationship with a partner of many years must be puzzled by the difficulty sex presents for many of their peers. Love and sex with the same person, who has travelled along the bumpy, difficult road of adulthood with you, is one of the joys and rewards of this age. *"In a long-term and loving relationship,"* says Sandra Paul, *"you've been growing older together and are used to each other's bodies. You know and appreciate each other and are comfortable enough with each other that you don't have to be perfect."* At this wonderfully accepting stage, when sex is part of the relationship, not The Relationship, it actually gets better. You can afford to be kind and generous to one another. You've invested a lifetime together and all that investment goes to bed with you.

In any relationship it's very little time before a lover's personality, character and quirks overshadow physical attractions, however splendid and lust-making. When your partner looks at you, it's not just the physical shell he sees but the whole you he's known and loved for years, quarrelled and disagreed with, been through difficult and joyous times with. The "you-ness" of you overshadows the finely lined eyes or soft tummy. Reflected attraction and love between two people conveniently blinds them to the physical faults, changes and imperfections of time.

Inexperienced and raw youth may be convinced passion fades, but in reality it only changes. The frenetic love of the early stages of relationships devours itself. It burns out because its oxygen is the newness and novelty of the body and its responses. But the end of this type of passion is not the end of a good relationship. Over a lifetime, a successful, passionately loving and fulfilling partnership is not one relationship at all, but several. You may be married to the same man but having your fourth or fifth relationship with him; as he changes, you change, and the ground rules, demands, needs, feelings – and sex – change too. It's this constant change within a constant framework that keeps couples together.

Passion deepens with age into something more than physical satisfaction. It is as powerful and as urgent, but has contentment, respect and solidity about it. To be with a man for the pleasure of his company and the way he enriches your life is more flattering to him, and more satisfying to both of you in the long term, than being with someone for his ability to make you walk differently in the morning.

Sex is an intense part of a relationship but it won't make a relationship on its own. *"As important as sex is, the long-term companionship becomes even more important,"* Pat Knight muses. *"When I was much younger and involved with someone else, I felt bored all the time we weren't in bed. The relationship dwindled away because we had nothing in common outside bed. As you get older you value the whole person. It's so important to be with someone who lifts your spirits, and you can trust.*

"Women always need a love in their life; knowing someone loves and cherishes you cushions you against the harshness of life." Despite youthful disbelief, familiar sex does not breed contempt, but comfort, the freedom to experiment, and licence to be yourself.

One of the most difficult situations women face in middle age is being suddenly single again, either through divorce or a spouse's death. Women re-entering the social and sexual minefield alone, after years with one partner, may find that although the game of seeking, finding, lusting and loving is the same as it was twenty years ago when they were last on their own, the rules are different. Early experiences make big impressions as one newly single woman explained: *"It's the difference between being touched with love and touched with lust. The first man I went to bed with showed no warmth or tenderness, something I'd taken for granted as part of sex for most of my married life. It's a huge and sometimes painful adjustment for women whose last date was a quarter-century ago."* Some women have no trouble plunging back into the singles pool at all. *"After the last sexless, miserable year of married life, I was wild to be free,"* says a recent divorcee. *"Men at a party were like a box of chocolates to me – I was looking for the hard centres,"* she jokes. *"It was getting rid of all the frustration and boredom of my marriage and I don't regret it."*

The suddenly single woman may find it difficult to meet eligible men unless work brings her into regular and natural contact. For most women at this age, the other men they know are their friends' spouses, definitely out of bounds. If you know what you want and don't fancy trailing around art

Sex

galleries or the Motor Show indefinitely, or are weary of well-meaning friends introducing you to "a wonderful man I know", you might join the ranks of women who have signed on with dating agencies and bureaux. The back pages of the most upmarket magazines have the most upmarket agencies, and if after the initial interview you don't feel comfortable with the agency, you're not committed to anything. Although women do advertise through the personal columns of newspapers, it's a more dangerous and unpredictable route to romance; an agency at least offers some protection and screening of other clients.

There is an etiquette in sex as there is in everything else; but this is one area where you shape the rules to fit your beliefs. Life without male companionship is dull yet women may be hesitant to begin a sexual relationship. They dislike and resent the criticism and disapproval of their family at the idea of their having "a friend", and may equally not appreciate the exuberant encouragement of friends who prescribe a sexual affair as "good for you" as though it was a dose of cod liver oil.

Nothing is more private and personal than sex, so your ethical code should be one you can live comfortably with, even if it offends your children, surprises your friends or goes against current morality. If it's right for you, it's right. Having established that much, there is a general consensus that any elegant sexual code of ethics must include discretion. However thrilled you may be to discover bliss with *him*, you simply cannot put up a notice at the post office.

Some married women find their sex lives fading away just as they should be moving into the richer, fuller years. A couple doesn't have to be passionately entwined every night to keep a sexual bond between them. It's kept alive with a touch, a hug, a hand to hold, a shoulder to lean on. But you must, and he must, be demonstrative, tender and attentive, even if only through the briefest of touches from time to time, a reminder of a passionate past and a promise for the future. Every long-term relationship sails into rough waters at some time, when the desire for one another is buried beneath myriad worries and pressures from the outside world. There are times of intense disappointment or sorrow, sometimes personal, sometimes affecting both of you, when you would rather not be touched at all. A certain amount of suffering or anger is better got through alone. But love is a living thing and needs to be cultivated to stay that way.

A large component of elegance is graciousness, and sexual elegance has the graciousness of neither forcing attention and affection when it's not wanted, nor denying it to a partner who seeks its reassurance.

Despite their advantages, renaissance women at times do feel threatened by younger women, just by virtue of their being younger. This is one of the heaviest sexual crosses to bear because although you can look sensational and love the way you look, there is a type of man who is always attracted to much younger bodies. Not for who they are but what they are: young. They represent for him all the qualities he's afraid of losing in himself. Youth to him is adventure, irresponsibility, energy and a carelessness too often confused with freedom. Women unlucky enough to live with such a reckless and feckless man suffer more than their fair share of self-doubt and pain. However, all women may be cheered by the words of a dashing fifty-year-old who openly prefers older women who are his contemporaries to the twenty-year-olds within his grasp. "I prefer reality with style," he says. "Mature women have a classiness that young women do lack. I also find even in just meeting, not sleeping, with women, that I don't remember young women as individuals, whereas something an older woman has said, or something about her personality, stays with me. They leave an impression."

It's unfortunate not all men have such taste and discernment. In mid-life a partner's infidelity can be particularly distressing if it triggers a crisis of confidence in a woman. Some women of course will merely find their husband's pursuit of youth in the flesh ridiculous and hope he grows out of it. But if you're one of those women who wants to know if your partner is or isn't cheating, here's how you can tell. You know your husband is having an affair with a younger woman if:

Sex

- ♦ He gives up glasses for contact lenses
- ♦ He says *"not tonight, dear, I'm too tired,"* and he's smiling
- ♦ He knows who Bart Simpson is.

An unfaithful husband may drive a woman into the beauty salon for a make-over, or into the bakery for buns and biscuits – *"food is very faithful"*, as a stressed-out and deceived wife said – or into the arms of a lover herself. These are all typical reactions. Infidelity never seems to be just about a spurt of physical attraction away from the home hearth, but unleashes a hidden agenda of repressed anger, frustration and discontent. In your greener years the first reaction was probably to either furiously rush out and sleep with someone, anyone, in retaliation, or throw the offending partner out in a rage. In youth, sexual infidelity is the one unforgivable crime, overshadowing personal black spots like selfishness, humourlessness, unkindness, thoughtlessness – he's allowed every bit of wild behaviour but wild oats.

Although the throwing out or retaliation options are tempting at any age, now you're older, wiser, mellower, and have more invested in your relationship than is possible at twenty or even thirty, you're likely to react differently, with more circumspection and subtlety. Every partnership is unique, of course, and every woman responds in her own way.

"I could not turn a blind eye to my husband's infidelity," says Frances Meachem. *"I'd fight to keep him, but I'd find it hard to forgive. I'd make an enormous effort to understand what happened though, where I would probably have walked out in my twenties. Now there are things worth saving, things we've built up together that are more important than a physical affair. I used to be very judgemental about people and their behaviour, but when you get older you see life isn't so clear cut, so right and wrong. It's one of the wisdoms that come with age, making allowances for people and their behaviour. It comes with experience of life."*

There are times, says Pat Knight, when you may know your man is having an affair, but you have a good relationship, and a long-standing one, in spite of it. It may be worth turning a blind eye to ensure the relationship, of more depth and importance than a fling, survives. Sometimes acknowledging an affair forces your partner to take action he doesn't really want to take, and does more damage in the long run. Many affairs, she says, are physical indulgences which blow over in time. They only become important if you make them important. *"It takes great maturity, strength and perspective to see that,"* she says, *"but the deep relationship of marriage is ultimately more durable than a fling."*

Occasionally, generating a little mystery acts as insurance against a partner's infidelity. *"It doesn't mean you have to have an affair yourself,"* explains Sandra Paul, *"or be coy or teasing, but it may be better for some relationships if he's not so sure of you all the time. Your partner shouldn't feel you're so predictable, reliable and unimaginative that there's no mystery and he can do what he likes."* In other words, every woman likes her partner to recognise that she is still attractive to the outside world and fidelity is her choice.

Faithless husbands should take note, however, that many accommodating women who turn blind eyes to their husbands' flings, agree that a discreet affair is a woman's entitlement too. No philandering husband should be so certain his wife isn't indulging in pleasure outside the marriage bed. Sex, like food, is one of life's best treats, and it's difficult to be on a diet all the time.

"I don't see anything wrong with taking a lover if you need to and nobody gets hurt, especially when a marriage is emotionally empty or has become a convenience, or you're both staying together for the sake of the children," Pat Knight says. *"If you're discreet and careful, why should you deny yourself? Life is full of experiences and you're entitled to some of them, maybe especially as you get older. I've heard older women talk so often of the affairs they* didn't *have, because of convention or their own hesitancy and fear, and what they recall most is the regret.*

"You realise as you get older that while it can be a great risk to your existing relationship, it can also be handled well, and the world won't fall apart. It's part of the 'life practice' older women have, and it makes them very attractive and

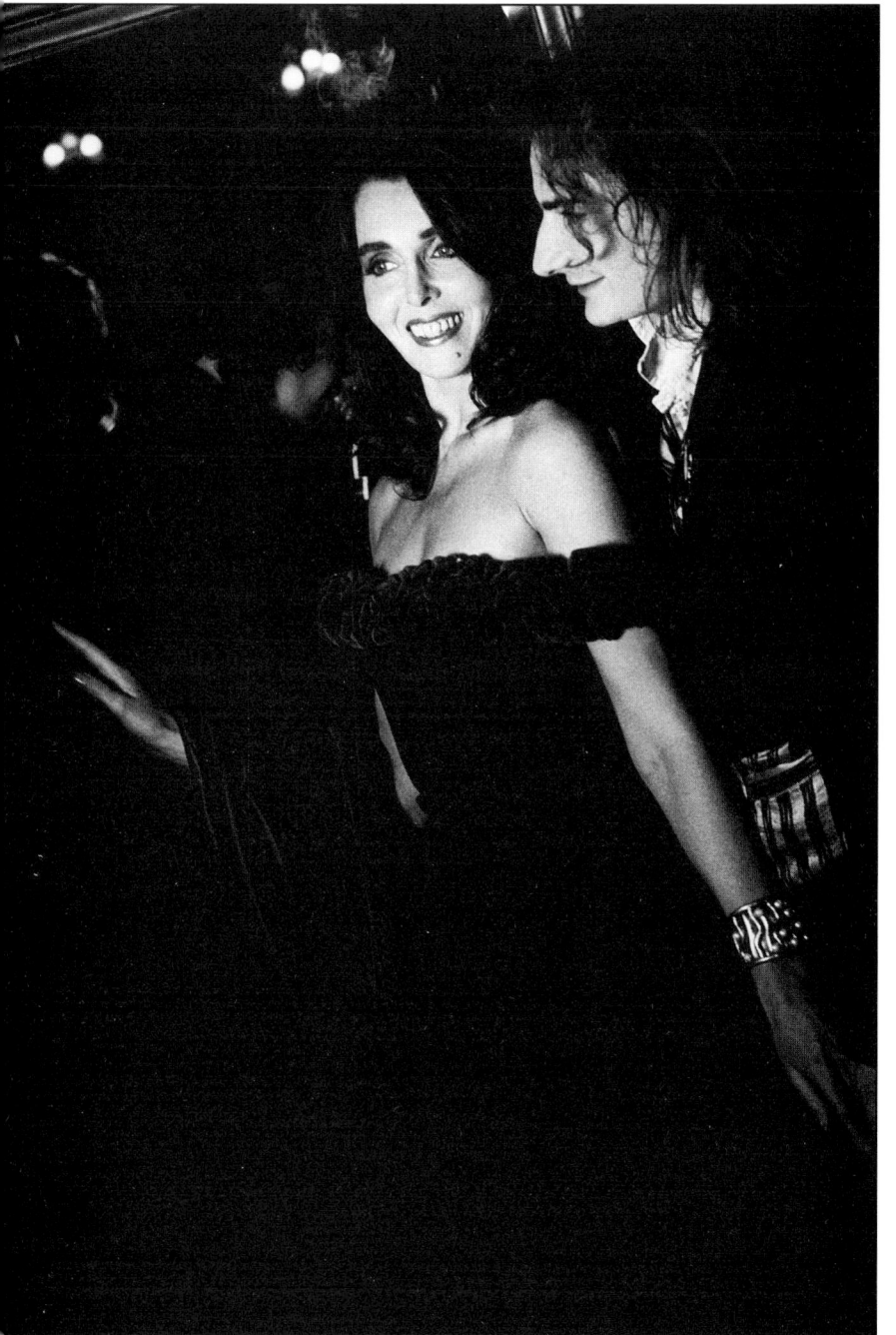

enticing to other men – this ability to look as though you could carry off an affair with style – which is something straying husbands might remember." Frances Meachem agrees affairs can be wonderful for the ego but cautions against the risk of discovery. *"You have to be sure you're willing to risk losing what you have,"* she says.

Many older women are. Accused by their husbands of losing interest in sex, they discover a surge of sexual appetite with a new man. If a husband is lucky he may get the overspill. Taking a lover is cheaper than psychoanalysis, healthier than gin and less fattening than chocolate, when it comes to beating marital mid-life blues. *"It's better than a face-lift,"* Pat Knight says. *"You can see what a lover does to a woman. I've seen women look younger, brighter, full of life and so much more confident. It's true what they say, that a little love becomes a woman. Knowing that you're desired makes you feel very powerful."* Other women echo her: *"A new lover is the best way to recharge confidence, self-assurance and pride in the way you look, and who you are, in your own importance and desirability."*

"I contemplate and sometimes do take a lover," says a very elegant woman. *"In my mother's day, she went out and bought a hat when she felt like this."* She didn't say how many hats her mother had.

No matter what age or shape, everyone wants to be desired and admired. Whether you act on the admiration of a new man is your business, but we all strive to inspire desire.

You can tell you're thinking of having an affair when:
◆ You wax your legs, not shave them
◆ You splash out on new underwear
◆ You start doing your old ballet exercises to stretch your leg muscles
◆ You see him across a crowded room and your mouth waters (only younger women blush).

You may hold yourself back from having an affair if:
◆ You need to lose half a stone
◆ You can't afford new underwear
◆ All those Jane Fonda workouts didn't work

Sex

♦ You need to lose half a stone
♦ You read the latest AIDS figures
♦ You need to lose half a stone.

There are several types of extramarital affairs. Some are a regular fixture of the marriage scenario, i.e. with a partner who doesn't see marriage as a curb or impediment to other physical relationships. Sometimes these are, or become, acceptable to a spouse: more than one woman has resigned herself to the fact that there are worse faults. He doesn't gamble, doesn't drink, loves the children, is a wonderful provider and probably also loves his wife, but women are his hobby instead of stamp collecting or golf. There are affairs which happen on the spur of the moment, a one-off that's as much a surprise to the perpetrator as to the injured spouse, and perhaps these are the most easy to understand and forgive by mature, generous partners, after the initial shock. There are foolish extramarital bouts of sex, that don't qualify as an "affair" – basically one-night stands after an office party or away at a conference, that have as much meaning and are rued in the same way as a hangover is. But what they all have in common is the ability to cause pain and real grief to a partner.

Anyone contemplating an affair should be very sure they know why they're doing it, what's at risk and whether they can live with losing what they've already got. Before escaping to a new relationship, if that's what you're doing, you probably owe it to a long-term partnership to attempt to save it: if you can no longer talk to each other, a clergyman, family therapist, or marriage guidance counsellor may offer the impartial mediation that two angry, guilty and hurt people can't.

In addition to physical affairs, there is a kind of mental infidelity too that both sexes indulge in under the approved label of fantasy. Everyone from sex researchers to agony aunts in women's magazines insists that sexual fantasies are a good thing and may spice up your love-making. But men and women are such different creatures, they fantasise differently. Men's fantasies tend to be coarse pornography of the "he-brutally-forced-her-legs-apart" type. Women's tend to be drawn-out romantic dramas, with a great deal of pursuit, often in historical costume – the "her-breast-strained-against-the-thin-fabric-of-his-greatcoat" variety. It's hard to know what's more inelegant, if fantasy slips over into reality, him calling you Madonna or you calling him Napoleon.

If stirring up your partner is more interesting than stirring up trouble, you must see yourself as a sensual, elegant woman; if you don't, it's unlikely he will. *"I stopped having affairs,"* confesses a happily married woman, *"when I realised how much effort I put into myself for my lovers compared to what I did for my husband. You know, a new man means sexy stockings and fresh perfume. A husband gets by with rollers at breakfast-time, no make-up on the weekends. I started dressing up for him and found I didn't need lovers any more."*

For all elegant women preparing for pleasure, the first essential is beautiful body care: scrubbed and scented skin, freshly washed hair, defuzzed legs and armpits, clean nails and teeth. Flannel nighties and jolly thick dressing-gowns do not suggest sensual abandon. The shops are full of delicious and enticing nightwear; if you can't afford it, wear nothing at all.

A good night cream that vanishes into your skin may be essential, but hairpins, clips, nets and anything else that makes you look like Giles's Granny has to go, or he will.

5 ♦ *Make-up and Skin Care*

Skin is the great traitor; more than any other bit of you it signals your age and gives away your lifestyle. The effects of smoking, eating, drinking, sunbathing, inadequate cleansing and pollution all show up on your skin, your life story exposed.

Skin takes the brunt of the assaults of world and weather. It's burned by the sun, chilled by rain and snow, made raw by the wind, clogged with smoke and chemical pollutants and dried out by central heating. It also adjusts to the kinder but unnatural assaults of perfume, make-up, over-scented soaps, powders and gels. It takes a great deal of manual abuse too – it's scrubbed, rinsed, pulled, wiped and generally gets more than its share of manipulation. At your age it's legitimately got something to complain about.

Women are terribly hard on their skin, Tania Mallet says. *"I've watched them apply moisturiser or foundation, rubbing it in so hard, working the facial skin like a punishment. If you treat your skin like a bit of old knicker elastic it's not going to spring back. Women should use very light upward strokes when applying make-up and use their baby fingers around their eyes. Good skin is so important. You can look better at our age with no make-up and a light tan if your skin is good."*

If skin is dull, grey and lifeless, any make-up, no matter how expert, will look flat. Good skin care and general good looks start from the inside out with a healthy diet – lots of fresh food and a limited amount of "poisons" like sugar, caffeine and alcohol. What you eat shows plainly on your face as you know when you look in the mirror after a particularly indulgent holiday or Christmas season.

Skin that once felt supple and elastic has lost much of its early dewiness by middle life, but it can still be soft and beautiful. Everyone's skin wrinkles and creases as they age, but the extent of the "parchment works", as one older woman calls it, greatly depends on genes and heredity, and how much unthinking damage you've done in the past, like baking in the sun or smoking heavily.

Whatever the sins of the past, you can slow down, though no one can stop, the ageing process but it's important to understand just what skin is and how it ages. Skin is the largest organ of your body, and often the most badly treated one. It constantly renews itself after wear and tear, protects the body and creates sensual messages in response to touch. It's not just one resilient, tough and attractive layer either: the epidermis is the surface layer which constantly sloughs off dead cells, allowing the young living ones beneath to form; below this is the dermis, home of the sweat and oil glands composed of collagen and elastin, tough tissues which break down with ageing; underneath that is a layer of fat which gives skin its plump springiness.

Women notice two things as they age: their skin gets drier and wrinkles form. Wrinkles are caused by changes in the deep layers of the skin as the collagen and elastin fibres break down, robbing the skin of suppleness. Dry skin is a sign of the skin's inability to hold moisture on the surface. There are two types of ageing although a woman looking in her unforgiving mirror may say, what does it matter, it's all ageing to me. You peer closely at your face and see the first fine webbing around the eyes, or notice the eyelids don't quite lift as readily and cleanly. Or the furrow between your eyebrows seems to have deepened into a trench. Self-inflicted habits like frowning may cause or accentuate the furrow, or a mouth pulled down at the corners.

Photo-ageing, caused by sun damage and other environmental factors such as pollution, causes more wrinkles than we need to have. In fact, the sun is the number one enemy of youthful-looking skin, causing deep wrinkling and drying out well ahead of the skin's natural lifetime.

Natural, or intrinsic ageing is the thinning of the skin, of

Make-up and Skin Care

which the fine lines which cover its surface are a visible sign. Many scientists now believe that we needn't age as early as we do, if we cut down on the ageing factors outside like pollution and sun damage. It's possible that pollutants trigger chemicals in the skin called "free radicals" which accelerate the natural ageing process. Some vitamins like A, C and E are thought to neutralise these free radicals and women are advised to stock up on vitamins, and eat plenty of oranges, wholegrain breads and green vegetables. Pollution can have a visible daily effect on skin. If you live in a city of any size, try wiping a clean white hankie across your brow at the end of the day – that oily greyish smear is the accumulated dirt, dust, smoke and car fumes eroding your fine skin.

You can't stop the ageing process completely and many wouldn't want to. A fine patterning of lines adds character and interest to a face. "You can see the person, not just the make-up," as a wonderful man says. However, dermatologists continue to come up with new skin-saving discoveries, to protect the skin from premature ageing. Many are now in commercially available products although you may feel you need a science degree to understand all these miracle ingredients. If you can believe the cosmetic claims:

◆ **Liposomes** are microscopic "delivery systems" which carry moisturising ingredients through the skin, not just leaving them sitting on top.

◆ **Nayad** is a substance that is believed to stimulate skin cells and put elasticity into collagen.

◆ **Antioxidants** are vitamins E and C which some dermatologists claim counteract and repair dry and damaged skin and promote healing.

◆ **Retinoids** are derived from vitamin A; the much vaunted and controversial Retin A is alleged to smooth out wrinkles and take years off a face. Originally used as a treatment for severe acne – its most famous client is Cher – it's supposed to penetrate the top layer of the skin and reach the dermis where wrinkles originate, smoothing them out. It is not without its drawbacks: although Retin A skin is smooth and supple, it is also ultrasensitive to sunlight, and may redden and flake easily. It is only available on prescription from a dermatologist or cosmetic surgeon.

Skin is often categorised into oily, dry and normal, but most women have a bit of all three or go through stages where one type predominates. In the broadest terms, skin that is easily chapped, feels tight and flaky, is dry skin which should be washed with a mild soap once a day and saturated in moisturiser. Toners and astringents can be given up. Oily skin has a perpetual shine or gloss, although most women's skin reflects this in patches or at times of stress, emotional upset or overindulgence. It needs to be washed thoroughly, especially when removing make-up, twice a day and wiped over with a good astringent. The closest women get to "normal" skin – clear, soft, unblemished – is by looking at young children. Some of these lucky children will grow into the select band of adults with clear, untroubled complexions but most will divide into the dry/oily/combination skin camp. The smoothest, softest bit of skin left to women at middle age is on their bottom: it doesn't suffer the wear and tear of the elements or exposure to sun that faces get and feels just what it is – protected.

Much is made of "sensitive skin" but all skin is sensitive in some way, in that it reacts to stimulants of weather, sunlight and cosmetics. Some very fair or redheaded women may find their skin reddens or burns more easily than brunettes and some women do develop sensitivity to some types of cosmetics or the dyes used, but every skin can be classified as sensitive when planning how best to care for it.

Many women give up soap altogether as they get older, considering it too harsh for their skin. Kari-Ann Moller, whose skin, stretched over knife-edge cheek-bones, certainly looks younger than her years, says soap dries her skin and cleanses with a solution, followed by moisturiser instead. It's true that some soaps can upset the delicate alkaline/acid balance of skin and some heavily perfumed soaps or those with a large detergent component can irritate it. Generally, avoid any soap that smells overpoweringly of Gardenias or your grandmother's handkerchief sachet: it's too perfumed. Skin toners, sold commercially to make skin feel extra fresh

Make-up and Skin Care

and squeaky clean, and a favourite with older women who feel they tighten the skin and close large pores, may help but some beauty experts classify them as non-essential. Filling the sink with cold water and emptying a tray of ice-cubes into it before immersing or splashing your face with it is breathtakingly refreshing and has the same shrinking effect on pores.

What skin cells need more than anything else to retain youthful elasticity is water. As you get older not only does your skin lose water, it also loses the ability to hold in the water it's got. Water is naturally a part of skin cells and most of it from surface cells is lost to evaporation, inclement weather and central heating. But you can put it back in. Women should drink six glasses (about a litre) of water a day to plump skin up, and use a good moisturiser. How much moisturiser? *"Buckets,"* says Pat Knight unhesitatingly. To lift that dry, dull look, exfoliating the skin by buffing and scrubbing to get rid of the top dead, dulling skin cells is a must. Most exfoliators sold over the counter are full of gritty grains for rubbing off the cells, but if you're short of cash a paste of oatmeal and water will work almost as well. Other treatments for dull skin are available at the salon: massage stimulates the circulation and "wakes up" lifeless skin as does cathiodermie treatment, a deep facial in which electric currents stimulate the face.

Don't forget it's not just the skin on your face which craves attention. A good rough sponge or body buffer should be used to get rid of every bit of dead skin on shoulders, elbows, thighs and back while in the shower or bath. Vigorous stroking sheds the dead cells and gets the circulation going.

Pat Knight's "buckets" of moisturiser all contain water, oil and some kind of humectant which attracts water and holds it on the upper layers of skin. These days good moisturisers have UV filters in them too. If it's beginning to sound more like a garage mechanic talking about parts for the car – *"hey Charlie, get me a couple of UV filters for the Volvo"* – you're out-of-date in the latest skin care musts, which now centre around avoiding overexposure to the sun, public enemy number one in the fight to preserve healthy, young skin.

Overexposure to the sun's rays is believed cause skin cancer

– there were an estimated 28,000 new cases in Britain last year. According to some experts, the risk of cancer is greater if you have lots of freckles and moles, or if you've been badly burned in the past. And incidents are much higher where there are breaks in the ozone layer, such as in Australia.

Until this century nobody who mattered wanted a tan. The pale, creamy complexions of Gainsborough's women or nineteenth-century Victorian heroines were a sign of their high station in life. They didn't need to go out and toil under the sun to earn their living: only gardeners, labourers and farm workers had brown skin. Women wore broad-brimmed hats and carried parasols to protect themselves from unseemly colour. During this century a tan has completely reversed its social credentials. Initially it was seen as proof that you could afford to get away to exotic hot climes and lie in the sun; a status symbol of better living. The tide of public opinion is changing though, as more is known about the sun's damaging impact. A light tan may be flattering, but grilling oneself to look like a leather monkey is definitely out.

Everyone out in the sun must use a product that filters out the most harmful sun rays. UVB rays are responsible for burning and the risk of cancer. UVA rays are thought to penetrate the skin and cause visible ageing through wrinkles. Suntanning products, and now many brands of moisturisers and foundation, are marked SPF, or sun protection factor, based on how long you can stay out in the sun and not burn. Obviously, the higher the SPF, the longer you can stay out, the greater the protection. For example, if the SPF is ten, you can stay out ten times longer than you could without the product and not burn.

If you always burn or tan with difficulty, the SPF should be at least fifteen; any product should be applied ten to fifteen minutes before stepping outside so it has a chance to penetrate your skin and maximise the protection. Regular sun-worshippers will probably already have discovered the body's more sensitive areas but they're worth repeating here. The tops of feet and tops of shoulders are prime locations for burns and often overlooked when slathering on the sun cream. If

Make-up and Skin Care

you're baring all, or almost all, remember your breasts will burn more rapidly than regularly exposed body areas like legs and arms. Swimmers need to remember that powerful UVB rays penetrate water, so swimmers need as much sun protection as sunbathers. Towels and sweat wear off even the strongest protective cream, so liberal reapplication is a rule too, not an exception. High protection cream is fine for most of your body, but your face and neck will benefit from a total sunblock. The neck is often the first part of the body to show signs of ageing, if lines ring it, from dry and sun-creased skin. Occasionally older women find that after a lifetime of lying in the sun it makes them nauseous and swells their feet and ankles. Their bodies have reached a point where they are literally "topped up" with sun, have had enough and can't tolerate any more. If you're a lifelong sun-worshipper don't despair: buy a wide-brimmed hat and a parasol, retreat from the oily fray on the beach and contrive to look pale and interesting.

When all the make-up and fake-up – creams, moisturisers, massages and clever lighting – just won't do it, and you find your face drooping ahead of its years, you may consider cosmetic surgery. Although dismissed with a line and a laugh by celebrities who sing its praises, going under the knife is never easy. Most doctors will tell you there's no such thing as minor surgery and the risks have to be weighed intelligently before submitting yourself to it. If having a new nose, or eyes lifted, or breasts altered is something you "think" will improve you, better think again. You have to be in no doubt that whatever the outcome it will be easier to live with than what you've got now. Why do you want it done? To keep an errant husband from straying? Because your best friend had it done and looks marvellous? Because you fear getting old because old equals unattractive in your mind? Your surgery won't change your husband's roving proclivities, your friend will still look marvellous, more marvellous than you perhaps, and growing old means growing better and into a new, richer attractiveness.

But, if you have a physical characteristic that is spoiling your enjoyment of life, sapping your confidence and holding you back, maybe cosmetic surgery is the answer. The first step is to find a reputable surgeon and take as long as you feel is necessary over consultants. It may be an everyday occurrence to him, but being physically altered is brand new to you. Ask every detail of the surgical process, and the recovery time: many women are unprepared for the shock of black and swollen eyes, numbness, or faint scars that remain after an operation. There are several types of plastic or cosmetic surgery, none are cheap, all carry some risk, and all involve an uncomfortable recuperation period; this is not a decision to make lightly or from the wrong motive.

Before actually submitting to the knife, many women's first taste of this combat against time is collagen injections. The collagen is pumped into individual lines and wrinkles, plumping them out and making them all but disappear. Although effective, the results are temporary, lasting about six months. If that's unsatisfactory you may move on to the big stuff:

◆ **Blepharoplasty:** If your eyes are droopy and heavy, and make you look continually tired and haggard, this eye-lift surgery may lighten your looks. Swelling and impressive black eyes are common after surgery.

◆ **Mammoplasty:** The breast is lifted upwards, reducing size and realigning the nipple. It does make breasts look pert and perky again but there may be loss of feeling around the nipple and faint, permanent scarring.

◆ **Abdominoplasty:** This is a tummy tuck, for overstretched skin due after pregnancy or massive weight loss.

◆ **Liposuction:** Often called body contouring, it involves literally sucking the fat out of the body through tubes, usually thighs, knees, jowls and double chins.

◆ **Face-lift:** Despite the risk of looking overstretched and skeletal, this is popular because it's instantly rejuvenating, lifting and tightening the skin all over the face. It can take as long as six months to recover fully and for part of that time your face may be numb. If you want to see just what it could do for you, suck in your cheeks and pull the skin back at the ears and jawline. Shockingly good, isn't it?

Make-up and Skin Care

While you're looking hard at the basics of good skin maintenance, nails and teeth should be included. Nails stand up to a lot of punishment: breaking and splitting from digging in the garden, scrubbing dishes and immersing in soapsuds and laundry detergents. They occasionally get crushed or squashed in doors just to pile the punishment on.

Nails are a good indicator of general health. A normal healthy nail is pink and relatively smooth. Small white spots may be normal but a whitish nail may be a sign of anaemia, a red-streaked one a sign of high blood pressure. Pinhole depressions may indicate psoriasis or eczema. Thick ridges, flaking or continual splitting indicates a shortage of some mineral in your diet, most likely iron or zinc. A persistent black nail, which has not resulted from an injury like dropping something hefty on it or being squashed should be seen by a doctor: it may indicate a tumour at the nail base.

Even without these dramatic afflictions nails can be in a pretty sorry state from neglect. A well-balanced diet is essential for strong nails as is using some protection like gloves when working in the garden or with harsh chemicals or detergents which dry the nail out. Good care means nails are kept clean, well-shaped and short, rather than long. Long nails tend to be weak and a well-shaped oval is more elegant than a curving talon.

It's worth a visit to a manicurist to get them started in the right shape and when following up at home, nails should be filed rather than cut and with an emery board not a metal file which can injure the nail. Cuticles, the curve of skin at the nail base, should be gently pushed back with a proper cuticle stick. Light or clear polish looks best for days unless you're dressed for an event – luncheon or a meeting or wedding – but in the evening colour can be as dramatic as you choose. Whatever colour, painting your nails is something that cannot be done in a hurry. It's not a pastime for the impatient and not a last-minute before-you-go-out-the-door thing either. If you decide to "do your nails" before an evening out, give yourself time to complete them, right up to letting the second coat of nail varnish dry properly. Many a well-painted woman has ruined her ten little masterpieces by hastily picking up her purse or pulling on a jacket before they were quite dry.

Toenails don't suffer the immersion in detergents or garden dirt that fingernails do, but they are too often squashed, flattened and mashed into ill-fitting shoes. Those narrow evening heels may be lovely but if they blacken your toenail they're never worth it. Ingrown toenails can be agony and require a doctor's care. *Always* cut toenails straight across and keep feet dry, especially between the toes, to prevent fungus infections which can affect nails too. Older women often find their nails get thicker and multi-layered with age and may need a chiropodist to cut them, especially the nails on the large toe. Clean feet, well-fitting shoes and socks, and a healthy diet all help keep nails in great shape.

Teeth take a bite out of your image too, if they're not well cared for. It's not just a sparkling white smile that you're after: major infections can start when teeth decay and the decay spreads into the body's bloodstream. One guarantee of poor oral hygiene is bad breath, an extremely inelegant feature. At your age you should always be following a healthy pattern of dental hygiene with daily brushing, flossing and regular check-ups. There is no reason for anyone in the Western world to lose a tooth to decay or gum disease these days. Regular brushing after every meal followed by flossing to remove the food particles a brush cannot reach, a fluoride supplement if there is none in the water supply where you live, and regular visits to the dentist will guarantee they last you a lifetime. Teeth are very tough: they tear and grind and chew, get pulled on by toffee and sticky fruits, and are often ignored or given a cursory brush. Decay is the result of sucrose manufactured by sweet things in your diet and although the sweetie brigade will point out there's sugar in apples as well as sticky buns, apple sugar (fructose) as opposed to bun sugar (sucrose) will not cling to your teeth in the same way.

Plaque forms on teeth as a hard scum and if not removed will get into the gum tissue and weaken the tooth. Gum disease is a major cause of tooth loss – bleeding on brushing, puffiness and sensitivity may be signs of it, and signs you're going to lose a tooth. Teeth need to be brushed vigorously, not just flicked over, preferably with a fluoride toothpaste, front, backs, sides and behind each tooth. After thorough rinsing, flossing dislodges more particles – if you don't know how to wield a length of dental floss effectively, ask your dentist or hygienist for instructions. If you want to check how well you've done, use a disclosing tablet, available from any chemist, to show up any remaining plaque on the teeth – it's likely you'll be shocked at the residue you've missed, but now you can see it (the tablet turns the residue bright pink or purple) you can clean it *all* off.

A woman poring over her skin for lines, wrinkles and blemishes will also find a lot of something else she doesn't want – hair. "I have more hair on my legs than on my head," moans one woman facing the summer season in despair. Unwanted hair on both body and face (and all hair on the body and face with the exception of brows, lashes and a neat pubic triangle is unwanted) must be removed. It is a thankless task. Like garden weeds, no sooner do you pluck or shave the offending growth than it starts pushing to the surface again. All women have a soft, downlike hair on their bodies; you can see it faintly around the hairline and jawline and more obviously, but not unpleasingly, on the arms. Unfortunately some women have a hormone imbalance which causes an excess of body hair to grow all over. These women need the help of a doctor, who may recommend an endocrinologist, a specialist dealing in hormonal disorders, rather than a beautician. For the majority of women, however, fashion dictates how furry they can afford to be. As the bikini line gets ever higher, the need to remove visible body hair gets more pressing. Electrolysis is the only method of permanent hair removal. It must be done by a professional, it's uncomfortable and very time-consuming. Although facial hair can be attacked in this way, the length of time to get results (by zapping the hair roots with electric currents) makes it impractical for legs and larger body areas.

Most women shave off body hair, despite the fact that it produces a coarse stubble very quickly, because it's quick, easy and cheap. As long as you use a good shaving cream or gel to soften the skin first, you'll get an efficient shave. Most beauty experts advise shaving in the direction of hair growth, down the leg from knee to ankle, for example. Fast and effective it might be, but shaving isn't the best method for getting rid of bikini-line hair unless you have a steady hand and nerves of steel. The angles are difficult and you may inflict some damage. *Never* shave your lip line: the coarse stubble that grows back will be far more difficult to remove cleanly than the original hair. There are other methods at your disposal.

♦ **Depilatories:** These slightly smelly, messy creams do a much better job than shaving at removing hair smoothly and cleanly. They're exceptionally good on the bikini line and lip line but you must follow the manufacturers' instructions and not exceed the time limit. Leaving the cream on too long can result in an embarrassing, red, puffy moustache in place of your original one as careless women discover. The cream contains a chemical that dissolves the hair and usually a soothing follow-up cream is included in the removal kit. When using a depilatory around the bikini line, don't do it in the nude: wear your swimsuit so you can see exactly how much hair has to come off, and where it has to stop before it burns or irritates delicate genital tissue. Most brands come with literature advocating a patch test first before full use, which isn't a bad idea, for a bad reaction to one of these creams gives new meaning to the expression "going for the burn".

♦ **Waxing:** This was invented, as any woman who's just had her first wax will tell you, by medieval torturers. Anyone who has not had a wax job before will likely gasp twice when the hot wax, and the strip of gauze embedded with hair is ripped from the skin. The first gasp is one of pain, but the second is one of pleasure, as waxing does make legs silky and baby-smooth, removing hair from a deep point under the skin near the root. Regrowth is slow too, another nice plus. Some brave souls attempt waxing at home, but you'd better go to a salon first, to get a feel for the procedure.

Make-up and Skin Care

◆ **Sugaring:** This is very like waxing, but without the pain, according to its adherents. Instead of wax a combination of herbs and sugar mixture is spread on the skin and sponged off taking the hair with it.

◆ **Bleaching:** This is more disguise than removal, as the hair will remain but be largely invisible. Many women prefer this method on the upper lip and unless it is extremely thick or coarse, the blonde light hair can be attractive. Home bleach kits are effective and easy to use so it's cheaper than a salon wax.

◆ **Tweezing:** Tweezing stimulates hair growth. It should only ever be used on eyebrows to pluck out individual hairs. Single hairs on your face or around a nipple should be bleached or snipped with scissors. Some older women are plagued by excess growth in their nose and occasionally ears; bothersome hair here should be snipped out carefully with barber's scissors. If you don't feel comfortable doing it, ask your hairdresser.

Having cleaned, buffed and bleached the skin to perfection, it's time to add a little colour. Nearly all women, whatever their age, benefit from a little unnatural colour. "Women," quotes Pat Knight, *"are not as young as they are painted."*

But they're none the worse for that. Cave-women no doubt daubed their faces with paints made from berries and bark. Roman women used vegetable dyes on their skins, mud and oils on their skin and hair; Elizabethans risked lead poisoning painting their faces white; the eighteenth-century *beau monde* powdered and rouged themselves liberally and sprinkled artificial beauty spots on cheek, lip line and breast. There's never been a time when some women weren't casting around for a little Art to help Nature. These days you can buy high-tech chemical compounds or "all natural" make-up – Kari-Ann Moller claims her organic make-up is so pure you can eat it. Make-up's purpose is not to radically change your looks so you peep out from behind a painted doll's mask, but to enhance your best features and correct or play down your less good. Clever use of colour, shading and outlining can enlarge eyes, reshape noses, hollow cheeks and plump out lips. Apply make-up in a skilful manner and it can take a decade off your face or bring out the true beauty of your age. Badly overdone, a woman can look like an escapee from the pantomime.

"Older women still have the bones but they've lost the bloom," Pat Knight says, "and good make-up brings that back." Every make-up routine begins with scrupulously cleansed, toned and moisturised skin. Frances Meachem suggests, to help your skin further, that you go one day a week without make-up to give skin a rest, and switch freely among brands so skin doesn't become oversensitive to one label. Many people suffer from sensitivity to make-up; it may be a particular brand, or more likely a colouring agent or dye. Sometimes, after wearing a cosmetic for years, your skin suddenly erupts. This kind of contact dermatitis is best treated by giving skin a break from the product, preferably with a non-perfumed, natural cosmetic. But "natural" and "hypoallergenic" on the label is no guarantee you won't still react; experimentation is the only way, or going without make-up for several days until your skin relaxes after its irritation.

Before you apply any make-up, you must have a good mirror in strong, clear light falling directly on the face, with no cross lighting. Assuming you're in a good light, clean and moisturised, you're ready to go: just as foundations support a building, so your face foundation is the base for all other decorative additions of colour and shade. Choosing a good foundation isn't as easy as it sounds. Most store lighting is different from home or street lighting and what looks like a warm biscuit tone in the store may look like greyish mud in the bathroom mirror at home. Older women need a light foundation with a tint of colour to give their skins a glow of warmth. Anything too light will look sepulchral. Too dark a foundation will make you look haggard. It's worth taking a friend along for a second opinion. Take a dab from the tester bottle or tube out to daylight or at least window light to see how the colour changes. Use your wrist skin as the testing ground, never the back of your hand, as it varies in colour and texture from your face. You may have to try a shelf full of brands before you find one you like for colour, density and

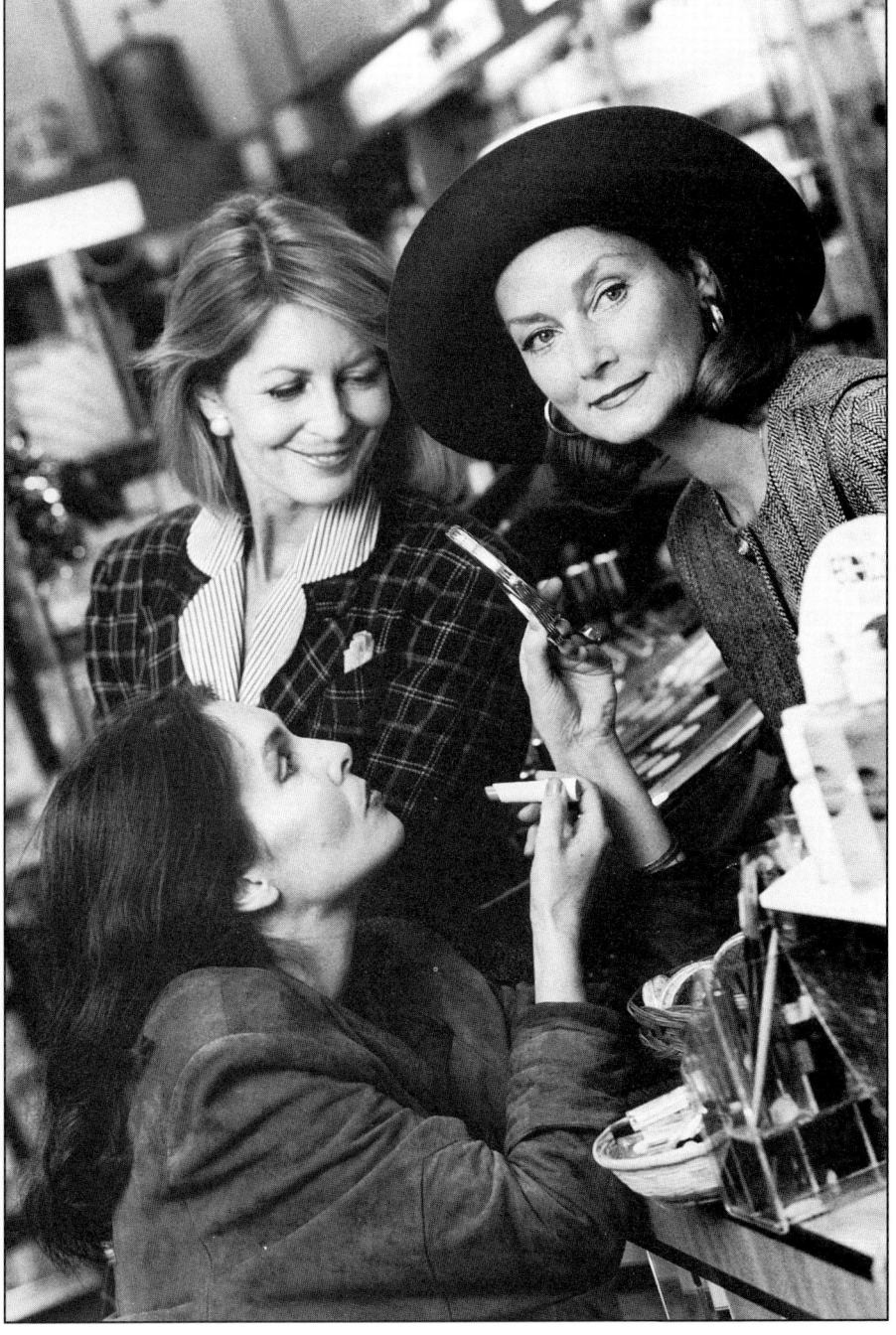

staying-put power, but it's worth it. Says Sandra Paul, "*you come to a cross-roads in your life as a make-up user where you can't wear the cheap stuff any more. You need to invest in good quality make-up. Foundation is always best applied after your moisturiser has had five minutes to dry. If the moisturiser's still wet, the foundation won't adhere properly and may streak or be uneven.*" Most women find it a good thing to put foundation on their eyelids as a sealant for a later application of eye make-up. Foundation should be applied with light, quick upward strokes and blended well at the hair and jawline so there's no masklike separation between face and neck.

Women don't necessarily need to use less make-up as they mature, but they do have to use it more skilfully. Youthful excesses, which looked dramatic and headturning then, look hopelessly overdone, even ridiculous now.

Peta Rogers, made up with a restrained and natural hand, sighs as she recounts the example of a friend who has failed to do the same. "*I have a lovely friend who looked a lot like Greta Garbo in her youth and she still makes up in the same way – except what was lovely and breathtaking in her youth now looks ridiculous. The make-up is all wrong, too extreme and overdone. Older women need a light touch. I think God does His best for a lot of people but they go against it.*"

Gone are the days, says Pat Knight, when in the height of the 1960s she used to wear three lines of colour with impunity: a pale turquoise shadow, an enormous brown socket and white on the brow-bone. "*I drew in big, wide eyebrows and wore amazing false eyelashes with individual false ones underneath my eyes. The effect was theatrical and very stunning. It took me forty minutes to make up every morning and those lashes were so heavy!*"

Kari-Ann Moller wore the Penelope Tree black-and-white look with this painted in eye socket and painted on lashes. "*I wore pancake make-up, false lashes, wigs, the lot,*" she says. "*I can't imagine it now.*"

There is a general consensus that one thing older women can't wear well is brightly coloured and pearlised eyeshadow. "*The pearlised shadow makes the eye look reptilian*

Make-up and Skin Care

because the skin is creased now," Pat Knight says. *"I think at this age, brown, grey or a shade one more intense than your foundation is most flattering. Bright blues and greens are very ageing and although pearlised is dreadful, a little luminescent colour can be good. Anything that throws back the light is youthful."*

Sandra Paul agrees it's a mistake to wear the brighter colours. *"Women now need to wear tones, not colours,"* she says. But you do need to experiment: brown can make your eyes look tired, but blue shadow needs a young wide-eyed look to go with it that older women don't have.

To dramatise all this colour and define your eyes, you can't wear too much mascara. *"Put on as much as you think you need,"* advises Pat Knight, *"and then put on some more."* Most women need the definition to bring their eyes out and eyeliner can be harsh and hard-looking. *"I have to wear mascara,"* says Tania Mallet with a grin, *"or my husband says I look like a white rat."*

The models agree that face powder must be kept to a minimum. It sprinkles and settles in creases on the face, giving it the cracked, aged appearance of an Old Master. Even if powder is used sparingly on the brow and cheek, it's best to avoid the fine lines around the lips and mouth. Powder may not be wanted but blusher definitely is. *"It's the one thing I wouldn't be without,"* Frances Meachem says. Pat Knight recommends a cream blusher if the powder ones sink into cheek lines. For an evening out and a really dramatic look, she uses a second opalescent blusher on the plane of the face just between cheek-bone and eye. All agree that brown and coral shades are more flattering to mature skin than the harsh blush-reds of ten years ago. Applying blusher is tricky. The effect should be one of overall warmth and glow, not startling stripes of colour. Apply very lightly at first, then deepen the shade. A healthy overall glow can be achieved by whisking a big fat brush laden with blusher over forehead, cheeks, chin and a touch along the nose; very enlivening, warm and rejuvenating. The bigger the brush the better – big brushes gently disperse colour naturally.

If you have grey hair it's doubly important to get some

colour on your face to give it life and lift. Deep but not garish colour on cheeks and lips counteracts the cool neutral impression of the grey.

Lipstick is another must. *"Faces look flat and dead without it,"* Frances Meachem says. *"There are hundreds of shades to experiment with so no woman can say she can't find something that suits her."*

A certain amount of experimenting about with matt, glossy, moisturising and pearlised tubes and pots is inevitable and not all of it a success for anyone. *"I really think women ought to keep up with modern make-up looks so I recently bought myself a bright scarlet lipstick,"* Frances says. *"My daughters wear it and I wanted to try it too – it might have looked wonderful, I don't know, but I do know I felt terrible wearing it. All night I was dying to wipe it off and put my usual coral brown colour on. I think it's good to try new things but you have to be prepared to let them go no matter how fashionable when you know they don't suit you."*

Says Pat Knight, *"You can go on choosing the same palette of colours: browns, or taupes, or reds or whatever because by now you probably do know what suits you best, but you can create a modern make-up look with those colours. Styles in make-up change like everything else: the shape of the brow, an emphasis on lips or eyes, pale or bright lipsticks. You have to adapt to the fashion."*

In addition to adding colour and life to a face, make-up can improve on the imperfections of nature. Shadow can open up deep-set eyes, narrow noses and hollow cheeks. Difficult complexions can be smoothed out in tone and texture by applying foundation with a damp sponge. Overall, no one will be able to see a particular bit of trickery; there's just the general impression you look finer, more "finished".

Cheeks for example: to hollow out chubby cheeks, first don't use pink blusher which fills them out. Second, suck in your cheeks and apply the blusher in sweeping strokes along and just under the cheek-bone. The cardinal rule is blend, blend, blend. The line between shader, blusher and foundation should be indistinct. You don't want to appear as a striped fugitive from *Cats*.

Make-up and Skin Care

Eyes not perfect? Small eyes appear larger if you line the outside of the top lid and under the eye in a very soft grey, either shadow or soft pencil. Deep-set eyes open up with light shadow on the inner corner of the lid gradually changing to dark shadow at the outer corner in an upswooping wing effect. Droopy eyes will lift a little with a discreet and soft line drawn from the corner and gradually widening out along the length of the lid. This is not the slick, black liner of your youth but a soft pencil effect perfectly blended with the almost matching shadow.

Lips, unhappily, shrink as women get older, so it's a good idea to use a lip pencil so you know exactly how much area to fill in. Very full lips can be made less "cushiony" by drawing the line inside the natural lips, but most older women will find the problem reversed: how to make thinning lips appear plumper. Deep coral colours fill out the lips and make them appear fuller than harsh reds. Sugary pinks are too pale and frail in an older face that requires richness. Although lipstick doesn't have to co-ordinate with clothing – unless, for example, you're wearing a brilliant red suit that cries out for bright red lipstick – lip colour should at least not clash or detract from other colour in your face, like blusher. *"You don't want to look false,"* says Sandra Paul. *"If I'm using blusher noticeably, I don't use too much lipstick, and if lipstick is commanding, not too much blusher. Deep colour is fine, but nothing too bright. There is a danger of overcolouring."* Many women get around the problem of a clash by using their lipstick as a cream blusher.

Cosmetics, as well as the faces and bodies they beautify, need sensible care too. Although they are formulated for long shelf life, once they do start to harden, flake, or the colour starts to separate, it's time to replace them. Like any substance they are liable to contamination by germs, dust and dirt. Keep lids tightly on and store in a drawer rather than a window-ledge exposed to light. Don't share your cosmetics with others, especially contact ones like mascara wands which transfer infection easily. In hot weather lipstick may "melt" a bit – you can keep it overnight in the fridge to preserve it. In very cold weather some moisturisers and foundations go on more smoothly if you warm them for a minute or two in your hands before applying. You need brushes for powder and blusher but although sponges and tiny brush applicators are nice for foundation and eye make-up, the best applicators are your own *clean* fingers. You can, if you're using Kari-Ann's all-organic make-up, lick them afterwards.

Elegant women cannot do without:	Blusher
	Lipstick
	Mascara
Elegant women have already binned:	Black eyeliner
	Shiny eye-shadow
	Copious powder

6 ◆ Hair

Just mention the word hair in a room full of women and the horror stories pour forth. There are very few women of any age who are happy with their hair and what it does, or doesn't do for them. It's always too long, too short, too thick, too thin, too lank and straight, too tight and curly, too grey, too mousey – hair is very "too", all of it impossible.

This is doubly unfortunate because hair is something you cannot keep hidden for ever, no matter how many scarves and hats you have, and it creates or contributes to the first vital impression people form of you. No elegant woman has hair that looks like it just emerged from a wind tunnel, is badly cut and hanging in her eyes or sticks out in a dry, frizzy halo around her head. Messy, unmanageable, unstyled hair instantly ruins a beautiful suit, destroys a glamorous evening dress and sabotages the most expert and flattering make-up. And women know it. Having your hair cut and styled at a good hairdressers is one of the greatest short-term lifts to the spirit known to woman. A woman's relationship with her hair does not improve with familiarity. After thirty, forty, even fifty years of coping with it, it can still be a difficult, awkward and intensely unstylish source of despair. True, hair doesn't have an easy time of it – from teenage years onwards, it's regularly assaulted to conform to the prevailing fashion. If you're anything over forty you've been spraying, teasing, dying, highlighting, perming, rolling, blowing, heating, pulling and tugging at it for more than a quarter-century. No wonder most mornings it fights back.

One way to gain back some semblance of control over your hair is to stop doing all those tortuous things to it as even gentle pulling and manipulating damages hair to some extent.

Healthy hair tends to be more manageable and is certainly stronger but bringing your hair back to healthy life requires patience. Like all outward beauty, its origins are inward. Dull and thinning hair may be caused by poor diet, or one especially low in B vitamins or iron. Your GP will be able to diagnose a low iron count due to anaemia and prescribe an iron supplement. Eating a well-balanced diet which includes eggs and wholegrains and taking a B supplement helps. Hair is often the last bit of you to recuperate after an illness, a lifeless, unmanageable reflection of your body's fight back to health. If you're going through a period of great emotional stress, that too will show in your hair's poor quality. Extreme stress or shock can cause a condition known as alopecia areata, in which large patches of hair fall out, leaving an area of the head totally bald. Eyebrows are often affected too. Rarely does it all grow back although a dermatologist or trichologist (someone who specialises in treatment of the hair and scalp) may offer some comfort; some drugs are thought to stimulate hair regrowth but are largely in the experimental stage and there are side effects. Women can take some comfort in the fact they seldom go bald in the dramatic way men do, but as women get older, their hair does recede at the hairline, thins and gets finer. Normal fluctuation of hormones in the menopause, or the stress of mid-life adjustment may cause hair to thin dramatically, although this kind of hair loss usually corrects itself when the body stabilises and general health improves.

In addition to inside influences, what happens to hair on the outside often hurts more than it helps. Vigorous brushing of the one-hundred-strokes-a-day variety may actually do more damage than good if it tears and stretches the hair. Gentle brushing and combing is healthier. Never brush wet hair; it will snap like overstretched elastic. Gently work a comb through it and use conditioner after shampooing to aid the comb's passage. Sun, sea and chlorine from swimming pools also have a disastrous effect on hair, drying it out and bleaching it to strawlike strands. Chlorine may affect the shade of coloured or tinted hair; blondes have been known to

Hair

emerge from pools with a distinctly greenish tint to their hair, so bathing caps are a must.

Hair that you're trying to pamper back to health starts as clean hair. Both scalp and the hair itself need to be free of dirt, oil, dry skin or dandruff. There is an ongoing debate about how often you should shampoo, with the "every-day" women threatened by dry scalp and the once-a-week shampooers by overstimulated oil glands. If you remember the heyday of voluminous mountains of teased hair you'll also remember that it teased up a lot better when it was dirty. Women left their hair a week or more between shampoos to get a more dramatic effect with the backcombing. After a few days' build-up, the oil, dirt and lacquer was truly monumental but it held the towering tufts in place. Today, it's better shampooed according to need rather than dictated to at the whim of a "look".

"Every woman has her own hair routine which comes after experimenting with what suits her best," says Frances Meachem. *"I wash my hair every day and since I've started using baby shampoo I don't use a conditioner any more."* Pat Knight is also an every-day shampooer. *"I went to a trichologist because I was concerned about my hair thinning, and he said to wash it every day to keep the scalp clean. It doesn't have to be a hard scrub, you don't want to damage the hair. I just slosh some baby shampoo through it and rinse very thoroughly."*

"My grandmother used to wash her hair once every three weeks and it looked wonderful," Kari-Ann Moller says. *"She'd think this every-day washing much too frequent. I admit her hair looked fabulous and I've tried to do it with mine but I just can't keep going. It goes through a horrible stage, and it looks really good as it starts to assert its natural self, but the horrible stage really is horrible. I've tried not using shampoo, just water, but that wasn't any good either. I think daily or frequent washing is a must for most women."* She harkens to some of her grandmother's advice though: *"You can make a brilliant rinse for your hair by boiling stinging nettles and using the liquid. It makes your hair incredibly shiny."*

Many women will be guided by their environment. If you live in a town or city, the amount of smoke, car fumes and other pollutants will make it necessary to shampoo every day; those in smaller, rural areas may find hair, like skin, lungs and everything else, stays cleaner, longer.

Hair is broadly classified into normal, dry, oily and combination type. At different times of your life it may switch from one type to another. Adolescents often have oily hair; pregnancy may produce the welcome surprise of suddenly fuller, more manageable hair; hair may suddenly become dry as you get older. Generally, oily hair – which is limp in appearance because of the build-up of oil – should be washed every day with a mild shampoo. Dry hair can be washed daily but only one lathering is necessary and a cream rinse or conditioner advisable. Normal hair can be washed daily, every other day, or once a week if it will wait that long. The aim of all good hair care is to intervene in its growth as little as possible or minimise the damage for what interfering steps you do take. Combination hair sometimes needs a two-part care programme. The roots which often appear oily need a good shampooing, the dry ends minimal. A little conditioner or cream rinse can be applied to the dry ends only.

Most important for all types of hair, is to rinse it thoroughly after shampooing, as though your life depended on it. Any residue left on the hair weighs it down, collects dirt, dulls the shine and makes it more difficult to style. If you can still feel a bit of soapiness close to your scalp when you lift your hair, rinse it again.

Sometimes all the things you've done to your hair over the years create problems: dry hair may be the result of overperming or colouring, not the hair's natural state, and the obvious answer is to abandon the damaging practices for a while until your hair heals. However, hair is a touchy subject because no woman feels she's got it absolutely right. Even women who have to look good professionally are wary about giving advice on hair. *"I don't think you can make rules about hair,"* Frances Meachem, whose own fair hair is actually a combination of highlights mixed with grey, says. *"No*

Hair

one is completely happy with what they do and all you can do is go on experimenting."

Despite driving women to distraction, no one can just forget about hair; it's too important to overall elegant good looks. "I feel most strongly that good hair lifts your morale," says Sandra Paul. "It's hard to feel good, never mind look good, if your hair is unkempt or needs a good cut."

Ah, the good cut. Like the holy grail, this wonderful cut that will flatter your face, easily shape your hair, and look the same after you shampoo it at home, reaches mythical proportions for some women. Part of the problem for older women is they feel limited by age: have they reached that stage where long or longish hair can't be worn?

"Long hair drags the face down a bit when you get older," Sandra Paul says, "but some women can look very good with it longer, especially when it's lifted at the sides with combs."

Kari-Ann Moller has worn her dark hair very long for years and doesn't contemplate changing it.

Short, soft styles are more flattering and make women look younger, Tania Mallet affirms. "You can wear it long if it's swept up and off the face. That's very elegant. But you have to have a strong profile."

"My hairdresser," says Sandra Paul, "and I totally agree with him, says that you should do exactly what you want when you get older. Why be dictated to any more? If you like it and it seems to reasonably suit your face and clothes and general style, why not have it any length you want?

"Men like long hair and usually get upset if their wives or girlfriends have it cut too short. It's an incentive for women to grow it, but you have to believe it suits you and be happy with it yourself." Women never outgrow the occasional urge to grow their hair, although usually impatience at the hair's normal snail's pace growth of half an inch a month leads to women abandoning the idea and having it trimmed up again.

Peta Rogers, who has gone to the same hairdresser for years, and claims she has the easiest hair in the world to manage when it's short, now and again decides she wants a change and will grow it. "I've always told my hairdresser never to let me grow my hair," she says. "Then one day I'll *go in and he'll want to give it the usual trim and short style and I say no, I'm letting it grow long now, and we'll argue, but I insist. Then one day I see it in a mirror at home, all higgledy-piggledy, and phone him up and say 'whatever are you thinking of, letting me grow my hair like this?'"*

Finding an elegant hairstyle is not dependent on money to spend in designer salons but honesty, says Tania Mallet. "You need to be able to look honestly at yourself, try something different that interests you, and admit it doesn't work if it doesn't," she says. "Being honest with yourself in the face of conflicting opinion from hairdressers or friends is very elegant."

The most obvious change women face at this time of life is going grey. Grey hair is not necessarily a sign of age: some women go grey or have a handful of silver threads from their twenties onwards. But even if you don't grey or whiten, hair colour, like skin colour, fades with age, and hair needs brightening up. Grey hair can be startlingly attractive on the right woman; on the wrong one it can be dramatically and frighteningly ageing as it straggles unkempt over a collar. "You do see women with beautifully cut and kept grey hair," says Frances Meachem, "and it looks wonderfully elegant but the key is to keep it perfect all the time. Anything less looks grubby and ageing."

Grey varies in shade too. That dull smoky grey is not nearly as riveting as a silvery grey. If you think your shade of grey has more in common with an old pillowcase than silvery snow, if you think you might be less than perfectly well groomed all the time, a little colour is probably a wiser choice.

There are several ways to get rejuvenating and lifting colour into your hair. Highlighting, done professionally in a salon, does minimum damage to the hair but brightens and enlivens it and is more subtle than an overall tint. If you're uncertain about the effect of an overall colour, try a temporary rinse or tint first, either at home or in the salon. These will wash out after several shampoos but it gives you a week or two to decide on the effect that colour has on your skin, eyes and wardrobe. Permanent colouring is best done by a professional in a salon. The chemicals need to be carefully

Hair

applied and timed rigidly. If you insist on trying one from off the chemist's shelf, read and understand all the instructions and follow them to the letter. A patch test for allergic reaction and a colour test on a strand or two of hair is also a good idea. The colour of the model's hair on the package is a guide at best. Most important, commercial hair dyes are for use on your head hair only: *never* attempt to dye brows or eyelashes; it could lead to blindness.

Finding a decent salon is a major part of hair crisis for most women, as is building up a rapport with a hairdresser. A salon doesn't have to be a high-profile, top-of-the-line place to do good work. Many women know, to their financial and emotional cost, that paying top prices is no guarantee you won't get a duff haircut. Often you're paying for the trendy location, designer décor and the fact the head stylist changed his name from Kevin to Nico. But some top salons deserve their reputations and if you have nothing better to go on, you might go on a friend or co-worker's recommendation. But be warned: *"Two women at work got marvellous cuts at this place so I went along too and it was okay but a week later I hated it,"* a not-so-lucky-but-typical woman confesses. *"It wasn't quite what I wanted, I couldn't manage the style but the stylist was determined to give me the look of the week and made me feel very out-moded objecting to it. I felt like a visitor from another planet."*

Older women are sometimes intimidated by what they see as "better" salons. They prefer the familiar comfort of salons in department stores or the local high street – which in both cases may be excellent. Or they may not be. Or a woman may just decide she'd like to try something a little more adventurous.

For a woman wanting to go a little more upmarket, the agony of approaching a strange and forbidding salon is almost phobic. Many salons do little to make older clients feel comfortable or welcome. There's nothing more disheartening than sitting, shampooed and dripping, in the old clothes you always wear to the salon (in case the chemicals from a perm or dye get on them) and wearing no make-up (it smudges or comes off with the shampooing, what's the point?) and seeing staff and clientele around you, dressed to the nines and young enough to be your sons and daughters. The "this isn't the place for me" feeling descends quickly. If you are hesitant and uncertain and question your "right" to be there, the stylist will know it and treat you with less respect. In really good salons this won't happen – teamwork between you and the stylist, in which you work with, not against, each other will give you your "look". But there are still too many salons around where the work on the hair is good but the customer relations fall down heavily, with staff mistakenly thinking it's part of the salon mystique to be snooty.

It helps if you're prepared for some intense scrutiny when you go to a salon; after all, the stylist has to look at you critically to judge what will best suit you. If you're dowdily dressed and unmade-up, he won't think much of what he sees. Nobody has to dress up to get their hair done but it helps not to look shabby. Pat Knight suggests women wear their full make-up when they get their hair done: it helps the stylist choose a cut and style that suits your every-day appearance.

It also helps to take a picture so the stylist has some idea what you're after. *"Can you fix this, I don't know what I want, can you do anything with it?"* is not helpful or encouraging to any stylist, no matter how brilliant. He or she doesn't know what you like, or don't like, what kind of work you do or social life you lead, what clothes are in your cupboard at home, whether you wear glasses, hats or scarves frequently, all things that reflect on the cut and style of your hair. Before you enter the salon, have some idea of what you want changed or improved. A shorter style, a fringe cut in, or worked out, a change in parting, a curlier perm, a different colour, streaking or highlighting – at least have thought about it enough to give the hairdresser some clues, and so you're talking the same language. After all, even the best stylist isn't a magician or mind-reader.

Survival at the salon depends on:
◆ Not being talked into a cut you really don't want; if you don't like the idea, assert yourself and say so, suggesting an alternative if you can;

Hair

◆ Not suffering unnecessarily. If your neck is breaking at the shampoo sink or irritating perm solution is dripping down your back, speak up;

◆ Taking a book to read if it's a long visit, such as a colour or perm; you'll have read most of the magazines already and a book will give you something to do other than make small talk;

◆ Having a supply of small talk ready, especially if it's your first visit, so you can feel more at ease with a new stylist;

◆ Not confiding your life story or the details of your messy divorce on a first visit; save it at least for the second visit;

◆ Tipping generously, unless it's the salon owner who's "done" you, in which case a tip is inappropriate;

◆ Not hesitating to return in a day or so if there's something you can't manage about the upkeep of your new style. Good salons never mind clients returning or dropping in for advice on how to manage their hair between visits.

Managing hair requires not only skill but the right equipment. Every woman should have a good quality brush and comb, blow-dryer, hot rollers and possibly a styling brush to keep their hair looking well. Never hesitate to ask your own hairdresser how styling equipment should be used, especially when new things, such as diffusers, come on the market. He or she will be glad you're interested and willing to show you how they work. If he or she isn't, it's time to join the great salon search again. No woman should still be using clouds of lacquer – it's hard on your hair, your eyes and the atmosphere. There are several gentle holding sprays and mousses available if you feel you must have something to support your style. The big question is what do you do with your hairdo at night? No elegant woman has ever admitted to using pins, nets, clips or swathing her hair in toilet tissue to keep the style, a big favourite in the bouffant days. There is a general consensus that it is more elegant to be tousled on the pillow and start afresh in the morning.

OUTWARD ELEGANCE

Do you have elegant hair?

Elegant Hair	**Unhappily Inelegant Hair**
It's strong and healthy, with high shine and colour	It's several uneven lengths, straggling over your collar, sticking out around your ears
You can run your fingers through it and it falls effortlessly into place	It hangs in your eyes when you bend your head
You wear it in a variety of neat styles	It covers your face in a wind, blowing around in untamed freedom, detracting from every outfit except, maybe, your jogging kit
It flatters your face, showing off your great eyes and complimenting your features	You're forced to tell people that Martians from space came down in the night, took your real hair and replaced it with this intergalactic substance.
Your loved one calls you "Kitten"	Your loved one calls you "Lassie"

7 ♦ *Clothes*

"Every woman has clothes but not every woman has something to wear."

Most women, discounting the exceptional few who found their style before forty and have been true to it, have cupboards and drawers full of unsuitable, ill-fitting clothing ranging from multi-coloured handkerchief skirts, to puff-sleeved blouses and stretch trousers. They lie or hang there, mute testimony to an utter lack of grip on your wardrobe. This is going to change. You've reached a turning point in your life when you need no longer be buffeted by fashions and fads, unduly influenced by what everyone else is wearing. You also make the eye-opening discovery that two good, expensive blouses are infinitely better than ten poor quality ones in dubious material. Fewer and better, quality not quantity, is the ruling creed for women seeking an elegant style. Clothes become increasingly important as you get older. A much younger woman can get away with a thrown-together look the way younger children get away with saucy behaviour and older children don't, but renaissance women benefit hugely from a show of elegance, taste and style.

Elegance in your clothes, says Pat Knight, is a reflection of your strength of character. It gives you authority and inner power when you know you look wonderful and look right. It says something about your judgement as well as your sense of style and greatly boosts women's confidence. A positive self-image automatically makes you more attractive to other people. Everyone is taken at face value at first, for better or worse, and if your image is one of style, confidence, taste and

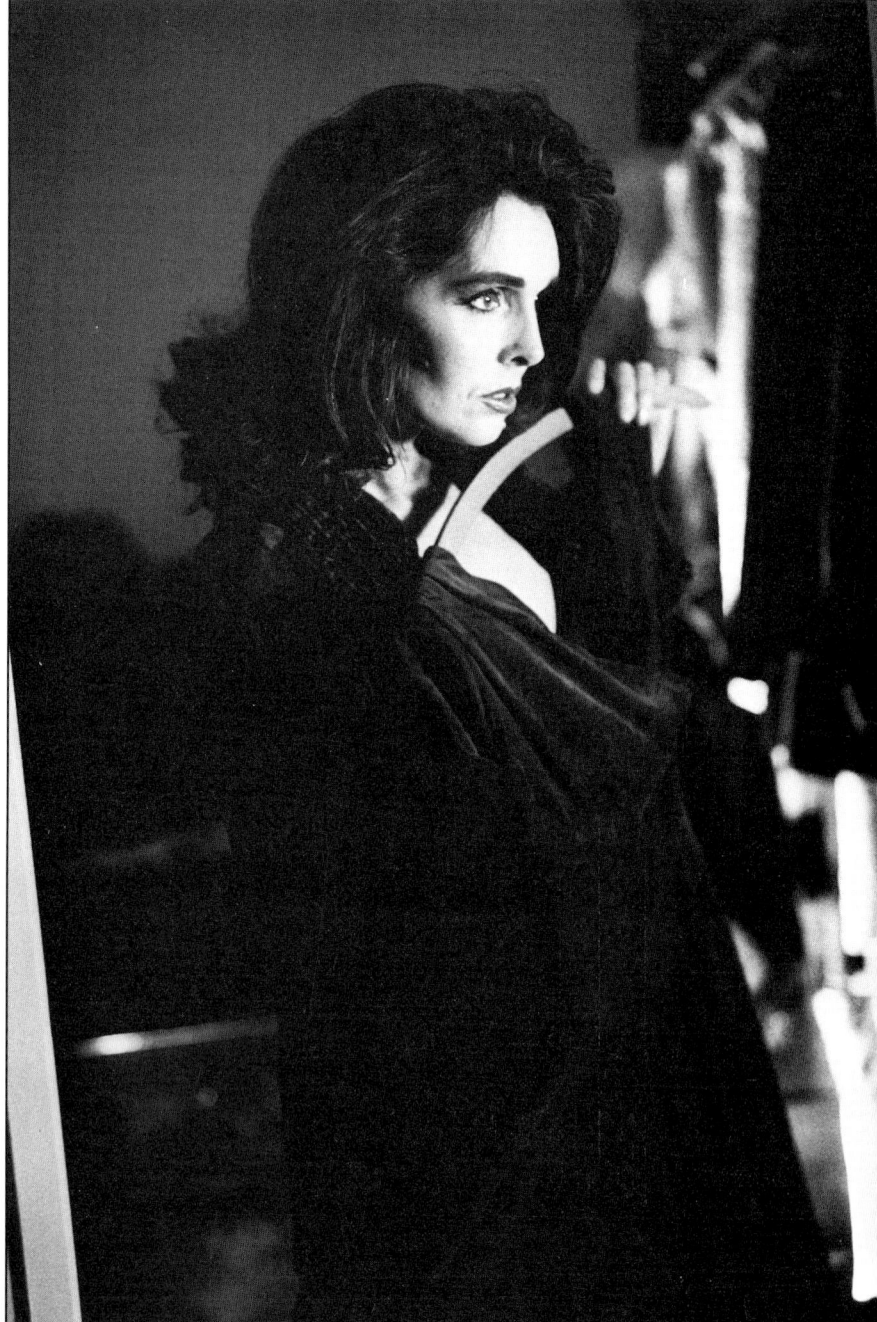

Clothes

judgement, that is how people will take you. Having said that, being totally wrapped up in your outward appearance and the quality and cost of the material on your back to the exclusion of other interests, is most inelegant.

A woman's clothes should be a source of pleasure and a way of presenting herself to advantage, boosting her self-esteem and enjoyment of being an attractive, sexy, accomplished, interested and interesting woman. Frances Meachem sums up neatly: *"You don't have to be obsessive about clothes but you do have to take them seriously."*

Women too often assume you need pots of money to be elegant, and buy everything with a designer label in it. Nothing could be further from the truth. Although money obviously gives you more choice and a wider field to range in, you can be stylish on a shoestring. Some women have an innate sense of style, and have had since their student days when a couple of pounds' worth of clothing from the street market could be carried off with the dash and *élan* that turned heads on the street. Other women have unlimited shopping money and still get it wrong every time. You can't buy a sense of style; it's an inward gift, but if you aren't born with it, you can learn it, although the process is sometimes painful.

Frances Meachem differentiates between fashion and style. *"Fashions come and go but style is something individual and more important,"* she says. *"It's the way a woman dresses to flatter her own taste and personality and express herself, and it certainly isn't confined to people with money. Dressing in top-to-toe Chanel isn't style, in fact it's frightfully boring. All it says is, I have enough money, or my husband's got enough money, to afford it. Lifestyle is a huge influence on style, but buying a 'look' isn't style either. When I had the boutique, there were customers who would come in and buy the entire window display, right down to the belt, hat and brooch. The customer got the fashion, but she didn't get the style. It's more personal than that."*

"There's a certain elegance in being confident enough to dress for yourself and not worry about what others think," Kari-Ann Moller says. *"That's how women develop style, being sure of what's right for them or putting their own*

individual stamp on passing fashion. You don't have to have the latest fashions if you've got style because you can carry anything off so well."

The confidence to wear what you like untroubled by the judgements of others is something women grow into, even the most polished and professional model. Pat Knight confesses to being so indecisive about what to wear for her twenty-first birthday party that she wore two outfits. *"I started the evening in a long pleated white dress and then changed into a green suit with a tiger lily orchid in my hair, which had been dyed pink! I made my second entrance at the height of the party, and I don't think many people noticed the clothes switch."*

"One of the secrets of style is putting old and new together, like an up-to-the-minute fashion item with an old favourite," Frances Meachem says. *"That look says a lot; you're still you in the same style, with an old favourite, but you've updated it with a new fashion. Your style remains essentially the same but subtly takes in new things, new ideas. Jean Muir, the fashion designer, has had the same style since the 1960s, but she always looks marvellous."*

Tania Mallet has strong views on style and has been definite about her look since an early age. *"I've always known my style and I haven't altered it since I started modelling,"* she says. *"The classic look was always me. Even in the 1960s I never wore Mary Quant or Laura Ashley. It just wasn't me, I knew it and avoided it."* Any woman who hasn't found her style by the time she is forty is in trouble and needs to rethink her approach to clothes and fashion, Tania says. *"Following fashion isn't necessarily stylish or elegant,"* she says. *"You have to take a long, hard look at yourself and decide what suits your figure, personality, the inner person you want to project, then stick to it. If skirts go dramatically up or down, you may alter your hemline a little, but the basic look remains untouched. The wonderful thing about classic clothes is that they never go out of fashion. There may be variation on a theme over the years but the basic classic style remains intact, and so does your image, your elegance."*

Clothes are a sort of social shorthand on display for other

Clothes

people to read you quickly. You dress to send messages to friends, lovers (current and potential), children, and colleagues at work. Your clothing says I'm responsible, I mean business, I'm capable and up-to-date, I'm sexy, I'm not interested, I'm relaxed and laid back. Clothes shouldn't say I give up, nothing fits and it was cheap.

You wouldn't go to a gala ball in sweatpants and overstretched baggy sweater and expect to be swept off your feet; you wouldn't turn up at a business lunch in an alarming all-but-frontless dress with a bottom-hugging hemline and expect anyone to take what you said about statistics and the economic recovery seriously. In less extreme terms, you send messages of good taste and confidence and liking yourself in a well-put-together outfit whether you're shopping or working, just as you send out a "don't bother me" message heading into town in an old skirt and rumpled jumper. If you think this aspect of clothes is frivolous, consider how all people, in all cultures, deck themselves out in their best finery on great occasions, whether they be coronations or a family wedding – dressing your best is a mark of respect in society, a point of personal pride, and the open knowledge that you know what to do, how to behave and that you belong.

Although style and taste are intensely personal, there are some things universally recognised as tasteless and without style. These include wearing jeans with white stiletto heels, knee-high stockings with a skirt, skin-tight trousers that advertise your panty line, and triple-frilled blouses à la mock Tom Jones. It is also tasteless and inelegant to keep flipping back the neck or inside of your jacket so everyone can read the label.

Today's renaissance women are liberated from having to don the "uniform" of middle-age as soon as they reach midlife. Says Sandra Paul gratefully, *"Clothes are so much easier now. There's been a revolution in how we think about clothes and what is suitable for women at this age. A fifty-year-old looks right in jeans if she's got the right shape. You have to make some concession to not being twenty-one: they have to be well-cut jeans and worn for example with a good shirt and a well-cut jacket, but there is very little you can't wear* comfortably and look right. If you've got a decent shape, and the confidence, the rigid rules are gone. The only thing I'm against older women wearing is short shorts. Little bits of you have been around for a while and are victims of gravity. But I don't see why you shouldn't wear a bikini."

A conversation about clothes is endlessly informative and insightful:

Frances Meachem: "You're never too old to wear anything you really like. These leggings that are fashionable now are great. I was looking at them for ages and wondering should I, shouldn't I, and finally my husband – a great believer in everyone looking their best and trying new things – said go on, why not? So I bought some and I love them, although I wear them differently than my daughters. They wear theirs with little tops, but I prefer at my age to wear them with long shirts and jackets."

Pat Knight: "There are no rigid rules about what to wear but body shape does change as you get older and you have to accommodate that. I love jackets and I love the look of jeans with a shirt and jacket. Some things are absolutely essential for women: a black jacket and black skirt, and a black dress. Sometimes the simpler the better because you can dress it up with scarves and jewellery or some stunning accessory. Women have to be careful with brilliant colours but primary colours are stunning, especially red. And white is wonderful because it reflects the light, which is flattering for older women."

Kari-Ann Moller: "I don't think women should have to tone down as they get older. There's a lot of talk about wearing neutrals and tones rather than strong colours and that's good if they suit you, but strong bold colours are also very effective. Age is no barrier. You can't dress for someone else, you have to dress for yourself and there is a certain elegance in being confident enough to do that. I like slightly eccentric older women, it shows such confidence."

Frances Meachem: "I buy fewer clothes now I'm older, but I buy better ones. A black skirt I bought and thought very expensive five years ago was a great buy because it's the favourite thing in my wardrobe and I wear it all the time. It's a big mistake to buy something just because it's cheap or on sale when it doesn't suit you or you don't really like it. I don't think it's necessary for women to wear neutral colours although I often do because they suit me, but some women look better in bright jewel colours. I do have a very vibrant yellow jacket but can only wear it on days when I feel confident and happy and outgoing. And I'd wear my bright yellow jacket with my good old black skirt. I never wear navy-blue though, it makes me feel like an air hostess."

Pat Knight: "You must have pretty, sexy underwear, it makes such a difference to how you feel. When you go out in your best clothes and best underwear, it promotes a sense of well-being and you feel ready for anything. When you feel attractive and at your best, other people are attracted to you."

Frances Meachem: "Probably the most useful bit of clothing I've got is a suede suit: jacket and skirt. Suede is great for the English climate, you can wear it all year round and it's very versatile for day or evening. I also feel every woman needs a little black dress. And I'm the sort of person who feels better dressed in tights, not bare legs, although sometimes wearing stockings in the evening is fun – they make you feel sexy. Things are so much better in that direction now – I remember those ghastly roll-on things with suspenders we used to wear! That's the best bit about being fiftyish now. Clothes are so much freer and we have such choice; our mothers never had such choice."

Kari-Ann Moller: "I've calmed down now a little about clothes. I used to be really outrageous and wear wild things. In the 1960s I remember wearing fluorescent pink boots, hot pants and tights and prancing down the King's Road. I was always putting on a show in those days.

"I still like clothes to reflect the way I feel and the actual feeling of the fabric is important to me. I don't wear synthetics. I love the feel of cotton, and silk. I'm very casual around the house, tracksuits and leggings – how else can you be with four sons at home, and cricket gear piled up everywhere, and I'm still doing the school run because I had my last two later, so my life is different from many women my age whose children are grown up. But I do love to dress up for the evenings or a party. I like to be sexy and that can be very elegant in the right setting. Elegance isn't the least bit prim, although a lot of people associate that with it."

Tania Mallet: "Looking back the only thing I really cringe over is platform shoes and those shorts with the heavy belt around the hips. They didn't do quite as much for one as they should have."

Sandra Paul: "I wore hot pants but with a cardigan down to my ankles as I didn't like the back view. And I loved the geometrical Corrèges dresses and wore them with white boots."

Tania Mallet: "Today I wouldn't advise dressing in too short skirts although miniskirts are in all over Europe. You have to follow fashion with discretion when you're older. The thing about clothes is that it's partly how you feel about them and present them. Sometimes you hate a garment but self-hypnotise yourself into thinking it's fabulous and your confidence goes up and you charge out to meet the world."

Frances Meachem: "I don't know if I'd wear something I hate. I've been known to get as far as the front door, then rush back and change; I have to feel really happy about what I'm wearing."

Pat Knight: "It takes some thought to organise a wardrobe properly. I keep all my bras, underwear and sweaters in see-through plastic bags, so I can see what's in the drawers at a glance."

Frances Meachem: "I'm very organised, my wardrobe looks like a shop. I never put anything away that needs cleaning, ironing or a button sewn on, or isn't ready to wear. That's a legacy from modelling in adverts where I wore a lot of my own clothes and things had to be ready on short notice. I'm a great believer in throwing things out. If you haven't worn it for two years, you're not going to wear it now, so throw it away. And throw out any shoes that hurt or anything with a permanent stain. I admit some things I've kept out of sentimental value or because they never seem to wear out. I have a pair of trousers I bought fifteen years ago;

Clothes

and a Hermès scarf that's twenty years old. I've never worn it but now it's come back into fashion."

Pat Knight: "Women get very whipped up about shopping. There's a lot of pressure to get out there and get it all right. I do try and get a whole look when I'm shopping, right down to the shoes."

Frances Meachem: "I found it very interesting to observe shopping patterns when I had the shop. There was a regular customer who came in who was a size fourteen and she always bought a size fourteen skirt and a size ten top. Psychologically she wanted to be a size ten. It's so important when you set off shopping to be realistic about yourself and what you're looking for. It's a great mistake to buy something one size too small and assume you'll diet into it. Most women don't. And be careful if it's cheap. If you're never going to wear it, it's not much of a bargain. I follow some rules when I go shopping. I try and shop on my own, always wear comfortable shoes, don't carry any extras like a heavy coat or umbrella, and if I'm making a day of it, I take a break and have a tea and something to eat."

Kari-Ann Moller: "Some dresses are contrived works of art. I had a wonderful designer dress that I couldn't move in. I love loose comfortable clothes so that's what I look for when I'm shopping. I buy quality because they're timeless and will last me a lifetime. I don't buy clothes for today, but for always. I buy classic things and then odd little trendy things and mix and match. I love to mix extremes like a really expensive jacket with jeans. I love to give myself time to think too; I don't like to rush into buying things."

Pat Knight: "Panic buying is always stressful and usually results in mistakes. I shop for summer in early March so I can keep calm and happy and shopping is a pleasure when the pressure's off. It's dreadful to feel you have to get something for the next day or for the weekend and be running around the shops in a panic."

Kari-Ann Moller: "I still get some of my clothes from jumble sales although the best markets are becoming too well-known to find really good things. At the other end of the scale I get some wonderful dresses from Jerry (sister-in-law Jerry Hall). But mostly I'm looking for clothes that are comfortable for me because that's a big part of elegance. Some of the old aristocratic families are elegant. They always look easy and comfortable and absolutely right, absolutely as if they belong, wherever they are. They have such ease of manner and they're never a top-to-toe matching package. Something will always be a little awry, a touch of the eccentric, an individual twist. That's so self-confident, it exudes elegance and it's that kind of relaxed, assured ease I look for in clothes. I do feel guilty about spending a lot on clothes. I've just bought a green velvet dressing-gown and red velvet gown, and I actually hid them, I felt so guilty. That's one difference between American and British women. An American would come in from shopping and say, 'Darling, look what I bought', and show it off; the British woman has to sneak in and hide it."

Pat Knight: "I rarely buy anything on a first visit to a shop. I like to see it and go home and think about it. Slim women can wear fitted clothes but plumper women should opt for soft, draping material, not hard-edged suit lines. When you're in the dressing-room, look at yourself in the mirror from all angles – including from behind. It can be quite a revelation. It's sometimes better to find a good shop you like and where you get to know the staff and the staff know you and will genuinely help."

Frances Meachem: "Big women often do go wrong when they shop. They buy baggy skirts and I think it makes them look larger. They probably feel smaller in them but it's a psychological, not physical reality. They'd look better in something more streamlined. Anything too tight is a disaster of course, or breast pockets on a large bust."

Pat Knight: "Most women are too careful when they select clothes. They go for a navy dirndl with a too short navy jacket, but they feel safe in it. I think it's a good idea not to stick to the guidelines of a lifetime, but experiment and try it all."

Frances Meachem: "Did we mention night clothes? There are some delicious night things around which every woman

Clothes

should have. I don't wear anything in bed, but if I did it would be sexy and lovely."

Enough eavesdropping on conversations about clothes? To recap: Six things elegant women will give up this year:

◆ Navy-blue box-pleated skirts

◆ Any colour box-pleated skirts

◆ Buying a piece of clothing one size smaller than you actually are because any minute you're going on a diet

◆ Buying one item in an alarmingly unusual colour because it was on sale even though it clashes with every other item in your wardrobe

◆ Buying anything that's a high-street copy of what the Princess of Wales wore last – you have to be young, blonde, thin, tall, rich and royal to carry it off the same way

◆ Buying anything the Duchess of York wore, ever.

For women who genuinely feel at a loss when faced with the racks and rails of choice in women's clothing, and are no longer certain what colours suit them now, there are colour consulting companies and wardrobe consultants who will advise you on what colours and styles to buy, and in some cases actually do the shopping for you. Some large department stores have a wardrobe planning service for their customers, usually professional women who want to look up-to-the-minute and chic but have little time to shop personally. Any woman can avail herself of these services, although they may not be cheap. Some colour consultants actually come to your home and swathe you in various shades and tints in the privacy of home. A quick glance through the Yellow Pages or your telephone directory will tell you what services are nearest to you; occasionally fashion magazines carry advertisements from larger or London-based companies.

PART II

INWARD ELEGANCE

Having paid such attention to the outward you on display to the world in clothes, hair, make-up and all-round presence, it's unfair to say that it won't make you elegant – but it won't. The outward picture is only half the elegant story. The inward view is equally important. All the finery in the world won't transform you into an elegant woman if inside you are crabbed and mean-spirited, selfish and dull, and out of touch with life around you.

Truly elegant women radiate a warmth and interest in others that marks their inner as well as outer quality. In the early days of her public life, that most public example, the Princess of Wales, was little more than a glamorous clothes-horse. She has become an ever more elegant woman because she has developed a style of reaching out and visibly caring about people; her rapport and ease with children, the elderly and the ill, her humour, interest and unaffectedness when meeting dignitaries or ordinary citizens shines through. It's her character, coupled with her clothes,

INWARD ELEGANCE

that make her elegant. The same is true in less exalted spheres. A beautifully groomed woman is little better than a doll if she doesn't communicate with, respond to and engage the people around her, if she doesn't exhibit the better side of human nature and the finer qualities of her own personality. She puts out her personal style to affect those around her; inwardly she is building up new interests and skills and deepening and enriching her personality. The following chapters explain what makes an elegant style and how to put it together and make it work for you.

8 ◆ *Personal Style*

Every woman has a personal style even if she thinks she has no style at all. Personal style combines your basic character and personality and learned and unlearned traits that govern behaviour and response in everything from intimate relationships to daily dealings with shop clerks. Manners are part of it, as are intelligence and temperament. How you handle yourself in all situations, whether challenging or mundane, is a test and revelation of your personal style.

Although personal style rests on the bedrock of your personality it evolves and changes, is added to and refined, as life and experience change and refine you. It's where elegance starts to form, because, as Tania Mallet reiterates, *"Elegance is never purely physical – it's outward plus inward. No matter how smart, chic or beautiful, you need grace, honesty and discretion and a givingness too."*

"Personal style survives and adapts to all your lifestyle changes," Frances Meachem says. *"It's the real you: you do change in some ways as you mature or get wiser or more experienced, as you grow out of some things and learn to appreciate others, but basically, there's a core that's still you. You can't remake yourself completely. Independence is a big part of personal style with me and always has been. I've been married and have children and those are deeply dependent relationships but me, personally, I've always felt I could do what I wanted. I need to feel I have the freedom to be more independent if I want it. That hasn't changed."*

Sandra Paul believes it takes women longer to find or grow into their style than men.

Kari-Ann Moller went through strikingly different life-

INWARD ELEGANCE

style changes before consolidating her present elegant style, although through every turnabout there's been the same strong need to feel a bit different, go her own way and keep the attention-getting edge.

"I left modelling when I was very successful at it to live in the country with my artist husband and two babies; then I completely jettisoned the hippie look and adapted a vamp look – wonderful, with bright red lipstick – and moved back to London; then I met and married Chris and was completely domesticated and had two more children and now I've gone back to modelling. I've looked so many different parts, but I've always had the same need to feel open to new experiences," she says.

Peta Rogers has approached life with a straightforward, no-nonsense style, partly because she never got round to making long-term plans for her life. Things just happened and had to be sorted out. Her parents lost everything in the economic crash of the 1930s, forcing her to leave school and look for work, and the Second World War made a mockery of long-term planning: one day at a time was enough. But in her many incarnations as model, publicist and editor, she always had the same direct and forthright approach. When a photographer wanted to shoot her for American *Vogue*, five minutes under his instructions in the studio convinced her that photographic modelling wasn't for her. No thanks, she said, and left. When a magazine editor asked her, then working in public relations, who should the magazine hire as the new beauty editor, she replied *"me"*.

Many individual characteristics create a style, like independence and directness, kindness, cleverness, spite, jealousy, diligence, compassion and impatience, but generally women divide into three broad categories in their dealings with the outside world: they may be aggressive, assertive or avoiding types of women.

To see them plainly, if simplistically, it's easiest to imagine them in personality-reflecting clothing. The aggressive woman wears a strapped-for-action unadorned severe suit that barks Authority. Or her aggressiveness may take the line of flaunting the most flamboyant and outrageous fashions possible, on the challenge-my-right-to-wear-it-if-you-dare principle. An assertive woman is less combative in her approach to life, adapting new trends but not forcing them on others. A woman who avoids situations may decide the fashion choices are too confusing and stick to a serviceable white blouse and navy skirt, on the grounds that no one could object to it.

Women who make a point of avoiding all confrontations and never or rarely put forward their selves, their ideas or needs, whether on the career or domestic front, do no favours to themselves or the people around them. It's unhealthy for others to feel they can constantly undermine you or assume what you need or feel is always of secondary importance. Whether it's your boss or your spouse who picks up this message from you, it's doing him no good and you harm.

Likewise, the woman who is abrasively aggressive is hurting herself, offending those nearest to her, and is probably not getting the results she wants either. Outright demands and accusations do nothing to persuade people to your point of view. Underlying most aggressive behaviour is the assumption that you know better how to do a thing than anyone else, not a view likely to be shared by others. Nobody likes to be ordered about constantly, whether they're your children, employees, fellow members of a committee, neighbours or friends. The message you send out is that they are forever incapable of making their own decisions or doing things by themselves or having a worthwhile opinion. Human nature is stubborn. If you order rather than ask someone to do something or stop doing something, they may dig in their heels and refuse.

A neighbour may have been on the point of stopping some drilling and hammering as he could see you preparing for guests at the barbecue but if you aggressively command him to stop, he'll make all the noise he can to work off his resentment. If you ask him politely to stop and explain the circumstances, he's more likely to give the DIY a rest. The same applies at work. Women recognise the difference between an aggressive and an assertive boss. On Friday afternoon with a

INWARD ELEGANCE

pile of work in front of you, an aggressive boss gives you an extra assignment with the curt instructions, *"just get it done"*. An assertive boss will get more work, more willingness and goodwill out of his employees by saying *"I know it's late, I know you're busy, but things have backed up at the other end, can you possibly get this out today?"* Elegant women spurn aggressive behaviour as it is profound bad manners. You can't have much of an elegant personal style if you're consistently rude, ill-mannered, negative and abrupt with others. It suggests a lack of consideration and unthinking selfishness that is far from elegant.

The most balanced personality is assertive – willing to speak up but not shout, more interested in finding solutions than aggravating problems, or ignoring them and hoping they'll melt away. Their emphasis is constructive not destructive. Both the aggressive woman – who suffers her own brand of insecurity and has to order rather than ask to impress her power – and the avoiding, timid, passive woman, need to learn to be assertive in a competitive and complicated world. Assertiveness is based, like so many fine qualities, on confidence. It's not the conviction of always being right of the aggressive woman, but a confidence based on feelings of self-worth. It tells you your opinions and needs are valid, and as important as anyone else's; that you too have a voice and a right for it to be heard. Women need this kind of sticking-up-for-yourself confidence when dealing with an angry neighbour, an unreasonable spouse, difficult children or obstreperous tradespeople.

The confidence to have faith in your opinions and the courage to voice your views, is a major part of personal elegance.

If assertiveness doesn't come naturally to you, you can invest in one of the many assertiveness training courses run for women at evening classes or by local women's groups or you can practise until it becomes second nature, rather like good manners. How often do you stop and think "I must say thank you"? – it's just automatic, ingrained good behaviour. The same is true of speaking up and out, firmly but not overbearingly.

Personal Style

For starters:

◆ Make clear "I" statements, along the lines of *"I feel we don't spend enough time together"* rather than vague complaints about the way a relationship is going.

◆ Specifics are very effective. *"I'm very unhappy about the bend in the new window"* is more pointed than *"It doesn't look much like the brochure"*, when confronting a tradesman.

◆ If it's criticism you're offering, criticise the behaviour not the person. *"Please don't leave your clothes all over the house, it makes it difficult for me to keep tidy"* is more likely to get what you want than *"only a pig would live like this"*.

◆ Stop apologising for things you haven't done. How many times has someone bumped into you in a crowded street or shop and your reaction is *"I'm sorry"*. Don't apologise for being there. You have as much right as anyone else.

◆ Say no when a request really is too great an imposition or will cause too much pressure and grief. You know your capacity and limits best. When you've done all you can and reached them, just say so and don't waste energy feeling guilty.

◆ Make sure your body language matches your words. Nervous grinning, hair pulling, shifting feet and clearing your throat do not indicate confidence and assertion.

◆ Always recognise the other person's right to be equally assertive and state their case. Two aggressive people locked in debate trying to gain points and carry the day is an argument. Two assertive people working towards a solution that will give both sides most of what they want, is a discussion.

An assertive attitude doesn't mean you always win everything, every time. You may fret that the solution isn't good enough, for anyone, that you could have done better, that maybe you should have tried harder in another direction. But, as Tania Mallet says, *"Part of elegance is recognising there are limits, to yourself and what you can do. I heard some wonderful advice: 'good enough is fine'. It doesn't* have to be perfection, whatever it is. Good enough will do."

Body language is as important as emotional attitude in telegraphing yourself to others. You send out signals every time you cross the room, hesitatingly, boldly, energetically, slowly. In close-up our body language intensifies. The pupils of your eyes dilate (grow bigger) when you're happy or pleased to see something or someone delightful, and contract when they see something ugly or off-putting. The low lighting in bars and night spots (which makes the pupil widen to admit more light) makes everybody look like they're glad to see everybody else which is why so many relationships that start at the bar have trouble surviving the cold light of breakfast. Eye contact is a big part of body language. Conversation calls for a direct gaze but break the gaze every few seconds or it will be too overpowering. Intense, unbroken staring happens only in moments of deep intimacy or aggression. Taking up space is something else to watch when you're working on your elegant aura. An elegant woman wants the people around her to feel at ease and comfortable; she doesn't stand too close to people she doesn't know well, regardless of age or sex. We all recognise a no-go zone around new acquaintances or strangers. Your daughter, friends or neighbour can stand considerably closer to you in a crowded train or bus than a total stranger.

There's a lot of body language in a smile too: a fifty-watt smile for the postman, one thousand watts for the most attractive man in the room. Most women recognise obvious body signals: arms crossed across the chest as a sign of fear or insecurity; sitting on the edge, rather than back, of a seat, indicating anxiety. When we're anxious we tend to touch ourselves reassuringly – winding hair around our fingers, touching or rubbing eyes or lips, all unconscious gestures that betray our inner feelings. Handbags, coats and parcels held tightly against you or over your arm as a barrier between you and the world look defensive and hostile, everything elegance isn't. Self-possessed women don't fidget, wriggle, chew pencil tops or pull their hair in new or tense social situations. If you're aware of giving yourself away with nervous habits you

Personal Style

can overcome them, not just for yourself but because they agitate and make other people nervous too.

"Elegance is an inner thing that gives you faith and trust in your appearance and character," says Kari-Ann Moller. "You can't sit there fidgeting in every new situation, it makes others so uneasy. It all comes back to self-assurance. Really elegant people are genuinely interested in others and not worried about themselves, so they don't feel uncomfortable because they've forgotten about themselves. They don't think 'how am I doing?' Other people's reaction is mirror enough.

"Women should stop trying to be perfect – elegance isn't perfection. It's letting the spirit come through. It's difficult to describe because then you're contriving it and when it's contrived it doesn't work. If someone makes you feel comfortable and they are comfortable too, that's elegant style; a nice, gentle atmosphere, though it can be exciting. In a person it's charm. In the home it means nothing stiff, nothing so perfect it intimidates people and they are afraid to sit down in case they dent a cushion. Ease, comfort, even languidness are better words for elegant style."

This emphasis on body language may sound one step short of reading astrological charts but it is significant. We all speak body language, whether we call it that or not. Correctly used it gives you control over your environment, at a party, in a new job or a crowded airport. It enables you to pick up aggressive or belittling measures others may be using against you and counteract them. It gives you power to be in control rather than always letting others control you, and that power gives inner pride and confidence to face any situation. If there is a single key to inner elegance it is confidence. You can dress in the most superbly elegant clothes, but if you scuttle into a room, eyes downcast, with shoulders hunched, you exude nothing but nervousness, insecurity, shyness and discomfort. Your discomfort is infectious. In those situations, people reading your body language will feel as you feel and be hard pressed to recall what you're wearing. Likewise, a bright and positive, warm personality can overshadow a less than perfect ensemble and leave people with the impression of an attractive person. When you walk into any place, whether it's

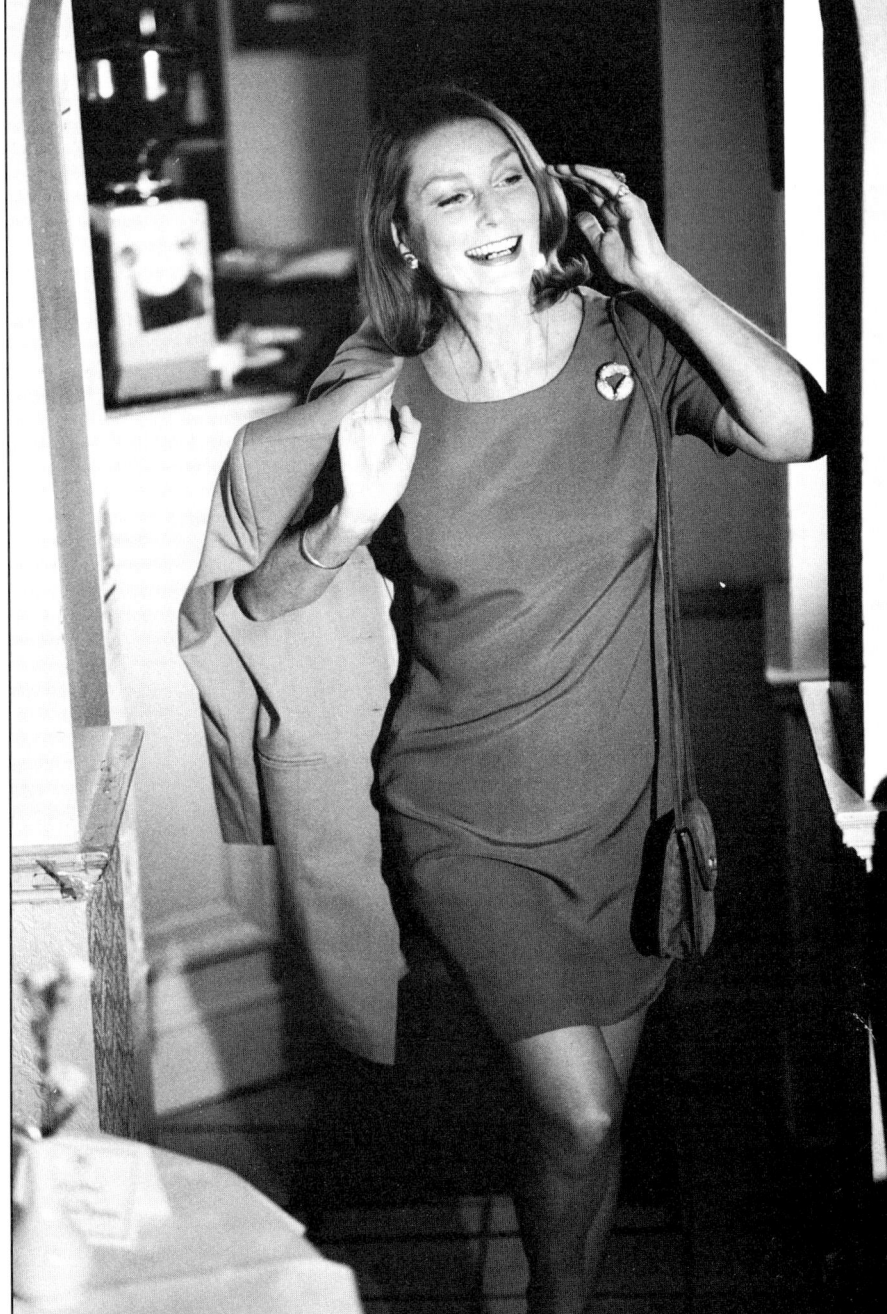

Personal Style

Sainsburys, sports day or the embassy ball, always walk in as if you own the place and expect that everyone will be pleased to see you. It's a kind of language everybody understands.

Personal style grows out of self-knowledge, when you know, understand and accept your limitations and flaws as well as advantages. It is developed by you, for you. You can't ape someone else's style totally and expect it to feel and be you, although there may be common threads running through the stylishly great and the greatly stylish. Style is not a series of strictures on behaviour but an opening up of possibilities so you, a worthwhile person, get the best out of life.

To prove your self-worth, pursue some simple sensual pleasures to reward yourself, boost your ego and reaffirm your value:

◆ Take a walk in the country, a hot bath, indulge in fresh flowers, listen to some special music or go to a concert. Do anything that reminds you that life, even your life, is not all work, commitment, stress and obligation. We're here to enjoy and enrich ourselves too.

◆ Take yourself off the waiting list for "Life". *Years* of our time are spent waiting for the perfect moment to do all the things we keep promising ourselves – waiting to finish school, to get married, to have children, for those children to grow up and leave home, for early retirement, for this, that and the other. The perfect moment never comes and a lot less perfect, but perfectly useful, moments go by while you're waiting for it.

◆ Recognise that being assertive also means being responsible; you have to take the responsibility for your actions and words. Stylish women don't drop their responsibilities; they don't take on more than they can honour either. That's where the assertive power of saying no comes in. If you make mistakes and are criticised for them, accept the criticism but remember you also have a lot of talents and positive qualities too. You are going to make mistakes, everybody does, but they are a reflection of what went wrong today, of tiredness, of bad luck, or a momentary thoughtlessness or carelessness. They are not a reflection of your worth as a person. Know it and believe it and others will too. Elegant women accept their responsibilities and their errors but they don't let them dent their belief in themselves.

Kari-Ann Moller remembers, *"When I first came up to London to be interviewed by a modelling agency in my country-bumpkin tweed suit I went into Fenwicks to have a coffee, and unknown to me at the time, all the top models took a coffee break there. There were several gorgeous, sophisticated models sitting around and I was so nervous, I spilt my coffee all over one of them; it was a ghastly and very inelegant moment."*

She recovered to take her place in the London modelling scene, but years later, emotional upheaval caused her to lose her elegant equilibrium.

"I used to drink too much socially," she candidly admits. *"I don't at all now, but there was a time when I knew if I drank I was outrageous and amusing. It was at a time in my life when I wasn't sure how I fitted in any more. I was back in London and socialised with the same crowd but I wasn't the same person exactly; I'd been living a different sort of life and become a mother and sort of lost my identity. I remember going to lunch at Jerry's [Hall]. I was a bit uncomfortable with her in those days. We had a lot to drink at lunch and afterwards we went out to a museum to see some clothes. When we got there I wanted to touch Queen Victoria's bed, so I climbed over the ropes and all the alarms went off! A guard came and asked us to leave and Jerry was really up in arms. She made me get into a taxi and told the driver to take me home, which made me more belligerent, so I got out and went into another pub. Everyone was just looking at me and I suddenly thought what am I doing? I went home on the bus and that was the last drink I had. It really shook me. The whole episode was a disaster but I quickly got my sense of self back again."*

Defining personal style is like trying to sculpt water; it rushes through your fingers refusing to take on shape or form yet is so recognisable when you come up against it. It's easier to define what it isn't – rudeness, tastelessness, lack of charm or compassion, gracelessness, overindulgence, jealousy, spite, cruelty – all have no place in elegant personal style. In defining a personal style, generosity and loyalty were key elements on everyone's list.

"*There has to be generosity and no mean-spiritedness in dealing with family and friends,*" Frances Meachem says. "*Confidences must always be honoured, whether between you and your partner, friends or children. Being interested in others is stylish because there's nothing worse than someone wrapped up totally in themselves. You have to be outward looking; too much introspection is unhealthy. Stylishness means being involved in the here and now, very current and not letting modern things defeat you.*"

Most women's style involves close friendships with other women, says Sandra Paul, especially as they grow out of the phase of seeing all women as competition and are confident enough to see them as allies.

Not all women are lucky enough to grow older with a close knot of friends around them. Changing circumstances, a divorce, a move to another town, retirement, disrupts many friendships and leaves women temporarily at a loss. There are myriad ways to meet new people and make friends at every stage of life: volunteer work puts you in contact with like-minded women of your own age, as do evening or day classes where you're all linked by the pursuit of common interests. University of the Third Age classes, a rather space-age sounding programme of very low fee classes on subjects ranging from playreading and literature to gardening, are ongoing in most towns for anyone over fifty. A part-time job, joining the local church, and going to neighbourhood events – a street car boot sale, bonfire night, jumble sales at local schools and churches, all bring you into easy contact with the people living around you. It takes time and perseverance for neighbours and acquaintances to ripen into friends but it does happen and it's up to you to take the first step.

Says Sandra Paul, "*Women friends are terribly important. Usually the closest ones live totally different lives or are at least in different businesses, so there is no competition and*

INWARD ELEGANCE

you can say anything in the world." You can't get away from the fact, though, that one feature of getting older is keeping tabs on how well everyone else is doing. In your twenties you look at your friends and wonder who they're sleeping with; in your fifties you wonder if they've had their eyes lifted, but of course have such elegant discretion you don't ask, and hope they'll confide.

Sandra Paul lists sensitivity as another ingredient of elegant style. *"You need to know when to talk and when not to. Discretion is important."*

Adding to your inward style from the outside world anchors it. Pat Knight takes refuge in the music of Mozart and Bach, which she describes as *"the epitome of elegance. I listen to them to relax and bolster my own equilibrium. It's reassuring to me that the human mind is capable of such heights; that when the world is so ugly and violent, to know human nature is capable of greatness too."* The lingering elegance of the music is a comfort.

A strong and elegant personal style is armour against the worst the world can throw at you and the slings and arrows of daily living. *"No matter what,"* an elegant woman says, *"I keep my belief in myself."*

9 ♦ *Spiritual Style*

In every woman's life there are moments of such intensity and deep personal meaning that words rob them of their richness. These moments may be created by great beauty, standing on a cliff-top at sunset; by complex and soul-sweeping music; by the birth of a child. They are moments when the intensity of pleasure, wonder and mystery combined lifts you from everyday life, even if only for a brief time. Deeply religious women may find it in faith; those inspired by natural beauty may find it in a garden; those awed by man-made beauty, in a gallery or concert hall. Whatever it is that so lifts and moves your spirit, it reaffirms two important things: one, that you're an intensely feeling, emotional being, and two, that you're part of something bigger than yourself. Something outside your self and your control can move and touch you. No matter what inspires it, this is your spirituality. Much of what inspires it is elegant and drawn from nature: certain birds and animals have a gracefulness we describe as elegant, as does much art, architecture and music. They all work on our minds and feelings. They all inhabit the world with us. They are all part of "our" spiritual elegance.

Every person needs a spiritual outlet in order to be lifted above the mundane and the ordinary; to feel there are still things to aspire to. Lofty as it sounds, it's a basic need to feel the world and everyone in it is capable of greater and better things, and to feel that you can see some pattern or make some sense of the world around you. We can't all be a Mozart or Shakespeare, Fonteyn or Pavarotti, or Mother Teresa. Some individuals are blessed with transcending gifts and

INWARD ELEGANCE

greatness. But everyone can do their bit, over a lifetime, to make themselves better, more attuned and compassionate beings and leave the world a better place, in however small a way, than they found it. That's real spiritual elegance.

It's not an overnight accomplishment. Spirituality grows throughout your life. And it is often in these middle years that women, reassessing everything from the length of their hair to their sex life and second careers, rethink their philosophical approach to life too.

"It wasn't until my children left home and started families of their own that I could see the continuity of life," a woman in her late forties said. *"I still feel young and energetic and yet here are my daughters, two more young women, about to have children of their own – the future seems very clear and I get worried about the state of the world. That's how I got involved in conservation and ecological issues. Not just because I want to breathe cleaner air, and all that, but because I can see in my own small family, the whole future of the human race unravelling. It suddenly strikes like a blow although you've known it, it's so obvious, and read and talked about it for years. But growing or grown-up children, to say nothing of grandchildren, make it real. You realise it's not just you alone in this world; the fate of one is the fate of all."*

Many women find their interest suddenly catches fire as they get older. *"One of the things you face up to as you get older,"* a woman explained, *"is that you're not going to go on for ever. It feels much clearer at fifty than at thirty. You want to be part of something that lasts. That's what drove me into these wildlife campaigns. If I could make some difference for the better, preserve something of the world as I know it for the future, then that is something of me going on for ever."*

Spiritual elegance is tied to this forethought and concern and interest in preserving better aspects of the planet, good things that endure and also serve a bigger purpose in a whole-world ecology. *"It makes you feel part of it, of all the world life,"* a woman says. *"It gives you a sense of belonging to something bigger than your own street or family ties."*

At the other end of the telescope, the intensely introverted

Spiritual Style

personal aspect is at the heart of spiritual elegance for women. *"Having a spiritual life is a very important part of being elegant because you have to have something on the inside in order to give something to the outside,"* says Kari-Ann Moller. *"Every woman wants to feel loved and valued. But the first rule is loving yourself – you have to love yourself first before you can love others properly. Self-love is part of spirituality because it is so central to the way a woman reacts to love. To what she is able to give and receive. It's vital to be able to do both. I find it quite difficult to receive. But I'm better than I was and I'm learning. There's an emotional exchange in any relationship and if you're emotionally or spiritually low, it doesn't work."* Or the burden is put all on one partner to the detriment of the entire relationship. Many women have experienced at some point in their romantic lives, loving someone who seems unable or unwilling to love them back. That hurts enough. But in some cases a kind of spiritual stuntedness prevents a woman returning openly and gladly and easily the love she inspires in others. She holds back for a variety of reasons, mostly protection against getting hurt or feeling too committed, or because she's spiritually empty and weak, never having learned to share emotion deeply. As many women know, but wish they didn't, giving yourself physically is easy compared with spiritual giving.

Not all of what is labelled spirituality is serious, high-minded stuff of great portent. Spiritual style depends too on the liveliness of your nature, and hanging on to some of the open, carefree, childlike (but not child*ish*) qualities that make life an adventure and a pleasure. Every woman, no matter what age, has a need for curiosity and some high-spiritedness, for enthusiasm and playfulness. Playfulness is particularly refreshing for the spirit. Women should never be afraid to show real emotions – real pleasure and real disappointment or pain. Freely expressed anger can be cartharctic; repressed resentment and frustration dwarfs your spirit. Real laughter is a tonic. Everyone should feel there's more purpose to life than just getting through the day. Some women seek spiritual life in retreats, in meditation, in new interests and new friends, or in old ones. However you seek it, it is the seeking, questing activity that does as much, if not more, good than finding your answer. Much of spiritual endeavour has no end, just because the subject is endless, for you and for the world at large. In great subjects like religion and art, you can reinterpret as you go through life but you can never know it all.

There are some things that will nourish and encourage your spirit along the path to discovery, fulfilment and understanding, and which will help you grow in strength and elegance.

◆ Take a break; as short as an hour, or as long as a week, go somewhere quiet and undisturbed, preferably out of your daily surroundings, to think about yourself and your place in the world. Many women have tried retreats, often run by churches or local women's groups, where they just wander or sit and think in appealing surroundings, undisturbed. They think, they feel, they relax, they reassess. The daily world is so rushed and noisy it is rarely we get five minutes for an unhurried thought when the world doesn't intrude.

◆ Feel pleased to be part of the world and a species that has accomplished so much. Despite all the destruction and horrors we're bombarded with, there is also much goodness and beauty in the world and the capacity (to say nothing of the need) for more is endless. Concentrate today on the best we've been and are, not on the grief and violence of the newscasts.

◆ Set out to discover how you can make a contribution, however small, to making things better for someone in your life, or in the world at large. Contributions don't have to be earth-shattering, just heart-felt. Reach out to the community or a world cause if you have the inclination: it does practical good and reinforces your feelings of being part of the universe and in your rightful place.

◆ Listen to your family and friends; not just with your ears, but with your heart. When your partner tells you his meeting went badly, he's also telling you "I'm hurt, my experience counted for nothing, I feel useless, I need to know you still love me." Your children may be angry

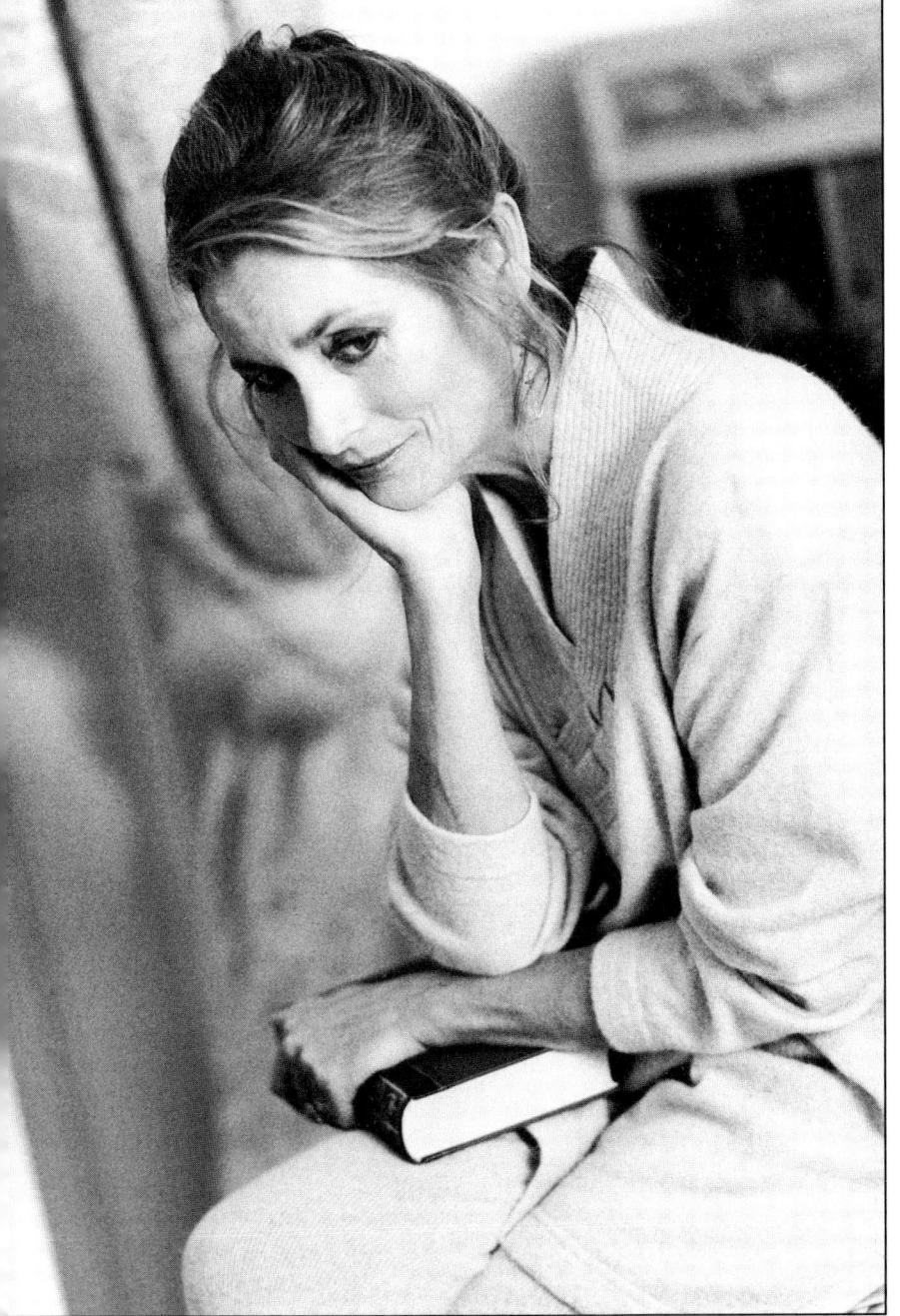

with you, even accuse or blame you for something that goes wrong in their life, but they also may be saying "this isn't what being grown-up was supposed to be like. I don't know what to do, help me." A friend joking about her husband's flirtations may be also asking for reaffirmation of her attractiveness and allure.

◆ Don't hold back generous impulses. Often you're on the verge of offering help or advice when a polite "don't get involved" policy clamps down and the offer, the kindness, the generous moment passes. Our "little, nameless, unremembered acts of kindness and of love" are an elegant sensitivity.

◆ Tackle a subject that interests you but which has never had enough of your attention. Whatever grips your spirit – if you love fine painting or music, are an avid reader or gardener – investigate your interest. It can only make it doubly interesting as it reveals itself. Take a course, read up on it, join a group that meets regularly to discuss this shared passion. It's not only good for your brain but for the inner eye or ear, and spirit too. If religion is an interest, most churches and synagogues hold study sessions through the week to discuss theological issues. It may not strengthen your belief, but it will strengthen your understanding.

◆ Commit yourself to something. It doesn't have to be an earth-shattering cause, but every woman should feel that what she does and how she spends her life is important, worthwhile and valued – even if it's just weeding the garden. Setting goals is very committing, as long as they're realistic ones. It lends a sense of purpose that just getting through the day lacks.

◆ Let other people be generous to you. Learn to accept compliments and kindnesses graciously. People need to give as much as they need to receive. Don't deny them their moments too. A compliment warrants a "thank you", not a simpering denial or brutish self putdown.

◆ The next time you think you're alone in an ugly and hostile world, go outside and look at the stars. Remind yourself you never know who's looking back.

10 ♦ *Skill Development*

Women love filling in questionnaires and surveys about themselves, for the very good reason they're convinced they have buried talents waiting to be unearthed that don't show on the surface. And they do.

There are obvious practical talents on display in careers and home skills, ranging from computer inputting and dentistry, to baking, decorating and gardening. But in addition to these visible talents, renaissance women possess a host of inner skills that may be applied every day on the career or home front that are taken for granted in a mature personality. Many of them are vital to career success, to running a home efficiently and to generally being happy and in control of your life. They are skills you can capitalise on whether you are at home, in the working world or have a foot in both camps with part-time or temporary jobs. Those skills or qualities include reliability, patience, loyalty, cheerfulness, moderation, optimism, open-mindedness and tact. They're skills that develop with time, experience and exposure to life in general, which make women your age rich in them.

These quality skills buoy a woman up whether she plans to pursue new interests at home for her own pleasure, upgrade her education, go for a career move upwards or consider re-entering the workforce after years away.

Let's consider a woman, one of a growing number, who is planning to return to work now the children are grown up, or grown up enough that she feels she can take on more for her own personal satisfaction; also, the woman who is forced to return to work because of financial pressure after a divorce, a spouse's redundancy or death, making self-support a must, not a choice. What holds these women back in an iron grip is lack of confidence; uncertainty about what's going on in the working world these days, fear her former skills are hopelessly out-of-date, timidity at mixing in with long-time working women.

Women's confidence is shaken because they're accustomed to thinking they've been "doing nothing" at home all these years. Actually, running a home and family requires many of the skills needed in an office or any organisation. Every situation you've coped with has cemented some sort of skill. If you have pulled a child's birthday party together, run a home, managed Christmas and holidays, there is nothing a working executive can tell you about planning, delegating, negotiating, budgeting, meeting deadlines, time management, decision making and stress. The executive may have been doing it in a wider arena and getting paid a lot more for it, but your skills and the executive's are the same.

Women considering a return to work tend to measure themselves against the technical and practical know-how of today and the last time they set foot in an office, before the onslaught of high-tech everything. But deeper skills, with which mature women are laden, are as eagerly sought after by intelligent employers as technical prowess. Learning a keyboard or which buttons to push is the easy part; but all the employee training schemes in the world can't teach a brash twenty-one-year-old the patience, dependability and cool headedness that living through a variety of crises for twenty years has bequeathed to older women. These personal skills – the ability to deal with crises calmly and cope with a variety of personalities – are real skills. As for the mechanics of the space-age computer, you can quote the middle-aged returner who countered her neighbour's query of *"would she manage"* the computer, with *"it's got an 'on' switch, doesn't it?"*

Women who have raised a family have plenty of experience giving instructions, solving problems and negotiating peaceful solutions to arguments. They have a lifetime's experience in explaining things, teaching, and lending a sympathetic ear, all highly prized qualities in new-style management, where

Skill Development

maintaining strong "human resources" as they call people is as important as working the technical side.

Because of these skills, women returning to work often excel in jobs where they have to meet the public or work in large offices where the hierarchy is not unlike the pecking order of a family. The scale is larger but the atmosphere is familiar. The very fact that you have been working on those skills which help people work together smoothly or make clients and customers happy makes you a desirable employee. Many companies are discovering that older women are ideal employees, whether they've been in paid employment recently or not.

Older women:

◆ have a strong work ethic
◆ tend to be self-starters, and are used to following a routine after years of running a house
◆ expect good service themselves when they're out, so they understand how important it is to give it
◆ are keen to take on responsibility, as they're used to responsibility of house and family and have the patience to see things done properly and not take short-cuts
◆ work hard for the company now, and are good role models for younger women in the company.

There are several job areas that women might match to their general skills.

◆ **Secretarial:** You will need up-to-date word processing skills. It is an excellent idea to start as a temp because it gives you a variety of office experiences in style, workload and the managing style of different bosses. It's very flexible, you can work when you please. Best of all, many temporary agencies provide free training on the latest office equipment. There are plenty of evening classes available too.

◆ **Sales:** If people are more attractive than paperwork, you may be an excellent saleswoman, especially selling in an area you're genuinely interested in. Many fashion shops prefer well-groomed older women who look dependable, trustworthy and get along with all sorts of customers.

They often have more patience than younger sales staff

in dealing with women hesitating over a purchase, and don't intimidate older shoppers with an offhand manner as many younger staff do. They may seem more knowledgeable too when selling items such as furniture or appliances. A twenty-year-old may look bewildered by the workings of a dishwasher but a capable, mature woman looks like she's been dealing with complicated appliances for years.

◆ **Teaching:** Many women welcome a return to teaching, although they may need refresher courses. It's usually possible to go back as a supply teacher or part-time to get your feet wet first.

◆ **Nursing:** Like teaching, a flexible career that women can return to part- or full-time although, like teaching, a refresher course may be necessary if you've been away from it a long time. Some women returning to nursing choose a specialist area at this time, now they're ready to think about a second career.

◆ **Counselling:** Women who are generally adept listeners, sympathetic and non-judgemental, make excellent counsellors at this age. They appear to the distressed both unshockable and practical. Their life experience gives them an authority that younger women lack. Training courses are usually offered by the counselling service, whether for voluntary or paid staff, but many women entering this field find a course of psychology from a local college or through correspondence courses gives them grounding and understanding in their subject.

◆ **Decoration:** Artistically inclined women may find that doing up a friend's flat leads to an off-the-cuff career as a decorator. Some women are blessed with a naturally artistic eye, and your taste and knowledge of fabrics and finishes may turn a hobby into the opportunity for a small business.

Wherever you feel your particular talents lie, now is the time to put them to the test. The more you do, the more capable you become, the more able to take on new tasks and the more your confidence blossoms.

While getting practical skills together is of prime im-

Skill Development

portance, don't neglect to boost your confidence by reminding yourself of inner strengths too. Even among professional women, the tendency is to list their skills as law, engineering, medicine, and ignore the quality skills of communication, negotiating, judgement and diplomacy.

Women never lose the need to expand their skills' horizons; the inner questing spirit of the early years is still there and now has time to dust itself off again. *"I don't feel drastically different from my youth; I'm still me, although a more experienced and wise me,"* says Frances Meachem. *"I don't feel incapable of doing anything although I would accept now there are some realistic limits to what I'm going to accomplish in my life. But I still have ambitions. There's lots more out there, more to discover, more people to know. You do change your goals as you get older, you never feel you've done it all."*

Not all the skills women want to acquire and develop in these years are for financial gain. Some women find they finally have the time to tackle an interest that lack of time and other responsibilities have made impossible until now. Of all the members of the household, a woman is the most likely to have shoved her talents and interests to the bottom of the pile over the years, making sure everyone else had a chance to indulge themselves first, partner and children alike. Now, it's her turn for serious contemplation of an activity or interest to enrich her life, and hone natural talent: painting, needlecraft, gardening, sports, politics, a musical instrument or learning Italian. Your skill at these special things that appeal to you is further affirmation of your self-importance and worth. Every woman needs to feel gifted and accomplished and recognised for it outside the security of her family circle.

Returning to university either as a mature student or through open university courses is another route for the self-achiever, and may lead to a revitalising second career. Whatever your skills are, home-oriented or career-oriented, brought to the fore by necessity or pleasure, it's vital to use them. Unused gifts tarnish – and all elegant women want to shine.

One of the great skills of living well is staying current and up-to-date in all things. This is your slice of history you're living through and you owe it to yourself to know all you can about the world and society you live in. The more you know, the more you'll understand, and the more you understand, the less you'll feel, as too many older women do, threatened by the changes in the world. Practising the skill of staying up-to-date is as important as a social skill, not just as a defence against an increasingly complex world. You're a more interesting companion and guest, more of a contributor to the world, if you can chat knowledgeably about the latest films and plays, novels, today's newspaper, about what people are talking about now in your street, your city, your country. Staying current opens you up to new ideas, makes you an interesting and informed conversationalist, makes you feel more alive. It makes you a participator, not just a spectator, in life.

None of these skills, for work or play, can be put into action and realised without a huge infusion of confidence. If, after all you've read, your nerve still fails you, here are a few confidence-boosting tips that will make you ready for whatever situation you're facing.

◆ Never disparage what you've done with your life so far, or harp on about how different things could have been if you'd done something else. It wastes energy and is totally unproductive. Everything you've been and done in life so far is good, even the bad, lazy, foolish things, because they've all contributed to making you the woman you are today.

From your mistakes you've learned all about what not to do. Instead of regretting them, call it experience and let it go. Honestly, you're the only one who remembers anything about it, everyone else has moved on.

◆ Don't compare yourself with others. Some may be outwardly more successful or accomplished but perhaps you haven't had time yet or the chance to show what you can do. Now's the time to put your skills into action, not sulk because someone else has done just that.

◆ Always look your very best. Trite as it may sound, when you're happy with the appearance, energy and confidence flood in.

Skill Development

♦ Don't try and do it all alone, especially if you're returning to work after a spell away. Get all the pre-job training you can, even if it's only reading the company manuals. Talk to working friends about their experiences and put the new job into perspective. At work, ask for help if there's something you can't figure out or don't understand. There's no crime in not knowing, only in not finding the answer.

♦ Be realistic. It's good for your confidence to do things really well, so give yourself a fighting chance. Tackle one part of a skill's challenge at a time, so you can enjoy it. If you're learning to paint, try oils not watercolours at first, which are much harder to manage. If you're going in for sport, golf will be easier than jogging. If you're going back to work, take a first job you can handle easily until you absorb the new atmosphere and not one that requires extra homework and night school to keep up. If you always set yourself unattainable goals, it saps your confidence as you always fall short of the target. Accomplishment, however small in the eyes of the outside world, gives a glow of confidence that can't be beaten.

Part of building confidence is distinguishing between yourself and the task when things go wrong. The cake you've been decorating may suddenly collapse – the cake is a failure but you are not. Even the most talented, highly skilled individuals face some failure in their lives. Great actors appear in dreadful plays or movies; writers write unreadable novels; parents of two wonderful children suddenly produce a third, a cuckoo in the nest impossible to manage. Their errors are a reflection of their personalities and judgement but also luck, often inexplicable. They are not signs of their failure as actors/writers/parents, and they are not failures.

Getting a grip on confidence is a bit like plunging into a pool. You can dither and fret on the edge and never find out what the water's like, or you can jump in – and suddenly find you can float, you're fine, you do have what it takes and confidence is keeping you buoyant. You need confidence to prove and exercise your skills and you need skills to boost your confidence. It's a merry-go-round but a happy one that's worth getting on because it builds up a better, more accomplished, more satisfied and lively you.

How to write a résumé/Curriculum Vitae
If you've been out of the workforce for some time, you'll probably have to submit a résumé or curriculum vitae to the company when applying for a job. Employers have a lot of reading to do, so make your résumé as brief as possible, and packed with information about yourself. If you don't type yourself get someone who does to type it up. If you're spared the résumé but given a standard form to fill in, make sure you complete it neatly and legibly and don't be shy about including personal achievements as well as your professional record.

A good résumé begins with:	full name, address including postcode, daytime telephone number, age
and goes on to:	last job *first*, position, responsibilities, salary, dates of employment, and on in descending order down to first job, including those part-time ones while still at school. It is appropriate to include a line about why you haven't worked for twelve years, i.e. because raising family
and then:	academic qualifications, with last school or college first, years attended, and degrees, also any extracurricular activities such as drama or debating society, and on down in descending order to primary school, including dates and places please
and wraps up with:	personal interests. Includes hobbies, second languages if any, clubs or organisations you belong to. If you're a returner after years at home, include any major community tasks undertaken, like organising a Brownie weekend or church or school fair. It shows initiative, organisational skills and willingness to take responsibility.

Skill Development

If there's room and you feel it's appropriate, a couple of lines about why you want to work for the company or why you think you're particularly suited to the job, won't go amiss. And that will do nicely.

PART III

TOTAL ELEGANCE

Elegance is not a quality that turns on and off like a tap. Once you've developed your natural elegance, cultivated it to full bloom, it becomes as much a part of you as your sense of humour or inborn temperament.

Since it's a central part of a woman, it touches every area of her life, in and out of her home, at work, at play, in her relationships with others and with herself. An elegant woman is elegant whether she is arriving at the theatre or digging weeds up in the garden; whether she is dressed in a shimmer of nightdress or for stripping wallpaper from the favourite room she's redecorating.

Keeping yourself outwardly elegant is hard work that requires determination and effort at first but it gets easier as it becomes second nature. Elegance feeds on itself – an outwardly elegant appearance breeds cool confidence, ease and assurance within; the inner grace applies itself to outward good taste and chic.

The result is always a better, more attractive and happier woman, looking and feeling her best, extending her personality to her surroundings and creating a wonderful atmosphere around her, the possessor of a positive and optimistic approach to life which warms others; she reaps the rewards of good friends and deep relationships with family and loved ones; her sense of self-worth and self-esteem encourages and enables her to fulfil some of her life's ambitions. The respect and self-love she shows for herself encourages others to do the same.

How total elegance spills over into all aspects of an elegant woman's life, we'll see in the next chapters.

11 ♦ *Homestyle*

Any woman's house, from a two-up, two-down to Buckingham Palace, is just a collection of bricks and mortar until she's made it a home. Homes give us comfort, shelter and privacy, an important privilege. They provide a central place for family and friends to gather, a sanctuary from the world. They satisfy deep needs for a place of safety, warmth and identity, and a place where you're never denied entry. So it's important that your home is as welcoming, pleasant and edifying as possible. A home is created not just by the furniture and furnishings a woman puts into it, but by the emotional associations attached to them. Renaissance women find that each room, whether it's the comfortably familiar ones of the last quarter-century, or the strange new ones of a new home, is layered with memories as soon as the furnishings go in. This chair moves into the sitting room and suddenly the room is coloured by the remembrance of the children embraced and read to in it; these long-stemmed glasses are unpacked in the dining room, linking it forever to the memory of an anniversary when these glasses were a very special gift.

Home is emotional for women, and central to their lives, as so many of life's crises begin in it, are brought into the open, and resolved, or not, in it. A home stacks up riches in the memory: parties, Christmas Eves, first days at school, major battles, quiet evenings with the children out, the day the ceiling came down in the bathroom, the holidays when a son brought home half his class to stay, the talks till midnight with a daughter who has returned to get married. Home is part of, and the repository of, family history, and a woman is usually the guardian of that history. Home means more to a woman than her partner. He may provide the building, but she makes it a home. She is in charge of it from the day she moves in, not just in the routine chores of organising and running it, but in creating a welcoming, comfortable base for herself and those around her.

As the emotional centre of the household, a woman creates the atmosphere, the principles, the house rules, that the family runs on. Although taste, needs and style change over the years, a woman makes the biggest impact on homestyle of anyone in the house. Whether this is through natural inclination or custom, it still seems to be as true now as it was in our grandmother's day. Although a woman has a full-time career outside the home, the home is still her territory; despite the demands of the outside world she is expected, and probably wants, to take on her second full-time job of organising and running the house efficiently and well, ensuring the domestic system runs according to her high standards. And although some couples share exact tastes and preferences in décor, in most households it is a woman who has the final say in choice of furniture, wallpaper, colours and the use rooms are put to.

The style the house is decorated in is less important than the atmosphere that pervades it. A woman needs a home that is warm and welcoming, attractive and pleasant to be in, and one that other people feel comfortable in. It is to some extent always a refuge from the world, a place to retreat to and enjoy herself in with family and friends. It is a place where she's likely to put the best of herself. Says Tania Mallet, *"All women furnish their nests as best they can. It's very individual. Houses are often an extension of a woman's personality. We're fortunate if we can have lovely things around us, but the things women treasure are usually treasured for their meaning, not price tag."*

Every woman wants a home that is as pleasing and individual as she is. Occasionally women fall in love with a "look" and import it into their homes *en masse*, or they may just get fed up trying to sort out styles and choices themselves, a rather end-of-the-shopping-day feeling. Entire houses are done over in country rustic with stripped pine furniture, right down to the loo seat, baskets and trugs stuffed with dried flowers artfully arranged in window seats, and a plethora of Laura Ashley wallpaper.

Others are rag-rolled and stencilled within an inch of their lives, with mottoes, vines and acanthus leaves sprouting around borders and corners in every room, like an ancient temple. Houses are awash in billowing Austrian blinds, with swagged and ruched material festooning every doorway, archway and window space. It creates more of a feeling of material gone mad and claustrophobia than elegance. Although these styles may all be elegant and lovely used judiciously in the right settings, a surfeit of one style in a smaller house tends to make it look more like a showroom than a home. In decorating, too much of a good thing often has exactly the opposite of the effect intended.

Women with strong personalities, who are sure of their own taste and decorate their homes guided by the same principles that apply to their dress sense and general approach to life, move with ease from one area of life to another. A woman with a pared-down look in her flat – sparsely furnished, with lots of off-white space and bare surfaces – may be reflecting her uncluttered, orderly desk at work, and her shaped and structured suits with little or no jewellery, all in the cleanest, hard-edged lines. Another type of woman may adore knick-knacks and a bits-and-pieces approach to decorating, filling shelves, counter space, ledges, tables and spare corners with curios, photographs and souvenirs. The look of random clutter may be no surprise to someone who's seen her cluttered and overpiled workspace, and detailed, bedecked clothing, use of jewellery and all kinds of fashion props.

For Tania Mallet, home has to be comfortable, rather, she says, like the clothes she wears. *"It's got to be smart enough to work, but livable in too. My dining room is attractive, rather than grand, my kitchen extremely functional. My drawing room emphasises comfort rather than designer impact. You want people to feel welcome, not awed and overwhelmed by their surroundings. In some houses you feel you can't dent a cushion; that's not nice for guests. It may impress them, or it may make them feel you're a nouveau whatnot."*

When some women talk about "doing up" a house, they usually mean a complete, themed overhaul, creating "a look", usually one laid out in an expensive design magazine. For the very well-off, or very canny, this is an option, but most women have to eat as well, and their decorating budget extends to paint, wallpaper, a spot of DIY, perhaps new carpeting and a few new purchases if they're lucky. A woman may feel she "isn't the type" that decorates, that repainting every few years is enough, and real decorating is for the well-off and leisurely. This is another myth that can be dispensed with at this time of life. As you grow in confidence and make a statement with your clothes about who and what you are, so you should grow in confidence and try something with a little more verve than beige, beige and off-white in your home.

Decorating need not cost the earth, and it is important – your environment influences your mood and behaviour, affects your personality and relationships. Dark, cluttered rooms immediately make you shrink inside, just as light airy rooms make you calm and responsive. No one is immune to the effect of environment so it's vital to make yours as much in tune with your personality and needs as possible. If you think you're unaffected to that extent by your surroundings just conjure up your response to being crammed in any city on a hot summer's day, and then strolling on an endless beach with the waves roaring in. Contrast the mental and emotional impact of the crowded tube at rush hour on Friday, and a deserted lakeside on a summer evening. Not just the place itself has its effect, but the colours, space, light, texture, shape and function of each place affects us.

All these combine in your home to produce an atmosphere that's pleasing or off-putting, stimulating or bland, relaxing or agitating. Colours, space and furnishings contribute most to your home's atmosphere.

A mix of colours and patterns can be pleasingly suggestive. Pat Knight decorated the bedroom and bathroom of a house that was next to a wood with wallpaper depicting exotic woodland scenes in differing shades of pale and dark green

Homestyle

with a few pink and ochre flowers scattered in the pattern. Curtains were green, carpets deep rose pink and the rooms and the wood outside blended together. *"The rooms and the wood threw back images of each other,"* Pat says. *"It was very harmonious, very restful. Room and wood were one entity."*

Colour

Colour surrounds us from the moment of birth, yet we all perceive it differently. Is a grey sea depressing or calming? Does a blue wall inspire you to think "clean" or "cold"? All colours affect moods, some drastically, so what colours you put where in your home requires serious thought. Although a colour can't have an actual temperature, people will swear that they are cold in a blue room and warm in an orange or red one. Yellow is thought to have an agitating effect: it's bright, it's sharp, a colour for when you're feeling on form, at your strongest. Pink, on the other hand, is calming, and in some correctional institutions, rooms are painted pink to diffuse the anger or violent feelings of prisoners.

There was a fashion several years ago to paint all walls in the house white or cream and add the colour through furnishings and pictures; it was safe and uncritical, but boring. Good colour, skilfully chosen, can do a lot to enliven and beautify a room, and paint costs a lot less than colourful rugs, pictures and ornaments needed to brighten and bring to life an all-white house.

Some colours are associated with life stages. Most babies' rooms begin in soft, glowing pastels, and graduate to primary open-your-eyes yellows and reds and blues when children start school. This colour scheme gives way to whatever the teenage mania is in their adolescent years – black ceilings, recalls a woman, who remembers her children's teenage colour scheme as even worse than the psychedelic pop-art styles of her youth. Parents relive their children's growth and development as they peel layers of paint and paper off, when they reclaim the house as their own.

Generally speaking, "social" rooms, the ones used for entertaining and gatherings such as drawing, sitting or family rooms, can stand the application of strong, bold colour, which wakes people up, is stimulating and lively.

A season or two ago, dark green was *the* colour for the dining room but its fashion is fading a little as hostesses discover that while it looks terrific on the walls, it can be unflattering to human skin tones unless the lighting is right – usually strong and bright and warm.

Dark colours are the traditional favourites for "serious" rooms like studies or libraries, perhaps because the sombre colours are conducive to serious work and tend to keep the frivolous at bay. Again, good lighting is vital if rooms aren't going to sink into gloom. Kitchens tend to get the light end of the colour spectrum because of light's association with cleanliness and hygiene; bathrooms are victimised in the same way – it's always white or something "off" – slightly off blue, green, pink, peach, everything very pale and wan. It can be pretty with the right accessories in place, but it's only convention and if you feel a silver grey and raspberry coloured bathroom could be carried off with style, carry on. Tiny "extra" rooms, a third bedroom or boxroom, that you've earmarked as your personal sanctuary probably *is* better decorated in peaceful, quiet, restorative colours, maybe with a touch of the sylvan in soft green and grey. Splashing out on bubbling primary colours, overstimulating reds and yellows, will rob it of its serenity and make it difficult to unwind in. Hallways and entrance halls are almost always coloured white or off-white; they may be considered a sort of household no-man's-land which belongs to everyone rather than the special preserve of one, so they are left with little personality. But everyone passes through or along them at some time in the day, and often a jazzy, bold colour brings them to life, especially in a small house, and lifts it with the kind of bright colour you can't put in a small room.

When you're shopping around for colours, don't dismiss one out of hand because you've never liked it. These days there are countless shades and variations. You may think you don't like blue, but you haven't seen the Wedgwood blue, periwinkle blue, robin's egg, arctic and royal, all repudiating your impression of blue as icy and dark. The myriad tones and

Homestyle

shades created by paint and decorating make the idea of "blue" meaningless. Some colours are more difficult to picture in their total effect and it takes a confident hand to use them. Green brings to mind gardens and woodlands and leafy foliage, making it a restful and pleasant colour, but used in abundance in a small room it can have a vaguely institutional look. It also conjures up other images besides trees. One great fan of green regrettably decorated the drawing room of her new flat in several green tones, imagining a languid bower effect, but admitted afterwards that it was dangerously like *"being under water. At certain times of the day, when the light hit the big wall, you'd almost expect a fish to swim past."*

There are more colours and shades out there than any woman can envisage. That's why many a woman has gone to get "some paint in a sort of peachy shade" for the bedroom, and returned to brood for days over chips and tester tins of "oriental ginger", "apricot cream" and "sun coral", dazzled by choice. Because of a colour's effect on the look of a house and the feelings of its inhabitants, it's worth taking all the time you feel you need to select the right tones. The unexpected in colour goes a long way to creating an elegant effect in a room. There's no gospel that says all four walls have to be painted the same colour and doing one in a lighter shade than the other three (or two and two) lifts the room and prevents the bolder, stronger colours you might love to use becoming oppressive.

As vital as the colour, is the light that shines on it, dulling it or bringing it to life. Colour looks different in strong or weak light, in sunlight or artificial light, at high noon or dusk, and changes with the seasons – the light cast in high summer has a brightness and quality that isn't there on a November afternoon. If colour is a major component of your decorating scheme you should try it out with different strengths of light, and you may have to alter the lighting in the room to get the effect you want.

In considering artificial light, kitchens need bright fluorescent lighting or the bright, hard, clear light of tracker spotlighting. Living areas of the house, drawing and dining rooms and bedrooms benefit from softer, diffused lighting, but there should be provision for the reader in every regularly used room. Nothing is more annoying, or symptomatic of inelegant planning or foresight, than to have rooms with poor light, so that you have to "peer" to see a newspaper or book, or hop from chair to chair, trying to catch the light. Good clear lighting is equally essential in the bathroom. Many women install dimmer switches in dining rooms, and bedrooms, so the lights can be turned down and the atmosphere, when appropriate, turned up.

Space
Most women's experience would be that all rooms in all houses are too small; that however much space is in an empty room, it's swallowed up by ever-growing collections of furniture, books and odds and ends. Although you can't physically increase the space, you can create an illusion of roominess or airiness by skilful decorating. Light colours on walls and ceilings open up a room and lend it spaciousness. Light doesn't have to mean boring and predictable creams and beiges. It can mean a blend of off-whites in shades of pale pink, peaches, greens or blues, even lilacs and greys, all of which will make a room spacious and pretty. Floor-coverings also play a part in increasing a feeling of space: bare floorboards, stained a light colour, tiles, or wall-to-wall broadloom don't break up the floor space the way several area rugs do. Rooms are often not so much small in dimension as badly designed, so the heating unit or extra door eats up what should have been a usable wall. Artful furniture arrangement may help, as will getting as much clutter off the floor as possible. High shelves, rails, or mantelpieces can be filled with treasures and won't impede physical progress through the room.

Furniture must be scaled to fit, which may mean the huge three-piece suite that fitted so nicely in your old front room may have to make way for two love-seats or a love-seat and chair in your new home. A "nest" of tables takes up less space and gives more usable, flexible table-top space than a single large slab of coffee-table.

Homestyle

In making any room elegant a prime purpose has to be to make yourself and others feel comfortable and at ease. Your home is an extension of your good manners; you wouldn't be deliberately rude to friends and acquaintances and neither should your house deliberately try to show visitors up or make them feel on edge or out of place. Relaxed and easy is elegant; stiff and overstuffed isn't. Some of the most elegantly furnished houses are filled with expensive, beautiful objects worth *looking* at, but the house itself is not worth *living* in; they intimidate visitors and inhabitants alike. Women who are used to the company of lovely things and value them for the sake of their beauty, tend not to fuss about them or show off. They're on display for the eye's pleasure, not the heart's envy. If you're decorating to display things you cherish and value, and if you want others to feel welcome and happy in your home and share your appreciation of these fine things, you are decorating elegantly. If you're laying out your private hoard, stopping just short of putting price tags on it all and restricting access to certain rooms or visitors under twenty-one, don't bother. Just as you don't need a lot of money to dress elegantly, you don't need a lot to decorate elegantly either. Well-thought-out colour schemes, comfortable and interesting rooms, a charming, open atmosphere, is real elegance, even in the smallest *pied-à-terre*.

Furnishings
If you have the money to indulge your superb taste and fill your home with antiques, Brunschwig and Fils fabric and original oils, you can assume you're putting together an elegant effect. But the obvious display of wealth blessed by the design guild is only one form of elegance in furnishing.

Elegance in the home operates on the same principles as elegance in other areas of your life; it depends on honesty and ease and the enhancement of the best you've got. Many women find that in their middle years they can start thinking seriously about decorating for the first time. Preceding years have been full of jammy-fingered schoolchildren, careless and boisterous teenagers and ink-stained students. The best decoration for the house was the toughest, most dirt and stain resistant, scrubbable anything. *"If I could have plasticised the walls and doors, I would have,"* reminisced one woman.

Now is the time, with children grown up or gone, for confidence in style to assert itself and for you to put your good taste into action. Once the principles and understanding of elegance are right, the rest naturally follows. A lot of the dressing with elegance sense applies in the home too: choosing a style of furniture that suits the shape of the room, choosing flattering, rather than strictly fashionable colours, buying fewer but better pieces, and being bold about mixing the old with the new, family treasures with expensive new acquisitions. A clever woman created an elegant effect in her elongated hallway by displaying a mix of original framed prints, a watercolour or two, and framed artwork from her children's schooldays. The combination of pricey and homespun was charming, assured and very satisfying. Likewise, good furniture can live happily cheek by jowl with "finds" from street markets, discoveries from holiday bazaars, and home-made results from crafts classes, if it's mixed and matched with daring and you like it. Collections where you least expect to find them have style and flair: one woman hung her collection of walking sticks and ornamental canes on her sitting-room wall; another hung antique farm implements picked up at country auctions in her hallway; another framed and hung her collection of beads, antique and new, in the loo.

A relatively inexpensive way to give a room a lift if you can't afford the floor-to-ceiling treatment is to replace cheap plastic light-switch plates, door handles and other fixtures with good quality brass, wood or porcelain ones. Expensive light fittings immediately make a room look better and may be money better spent than on a decorator. The very well-off can afford to have an interior decorator come in and "do" their house, but like buying a designer suit, it says only that you have the money to pay his bill, not that it's right for the house or you, or that you even like it. It can be more honest, more elegant, to create your own look and reflect yourself more truly. Your look may not be able to say *"it took a design team six months to put this together"* but most people would

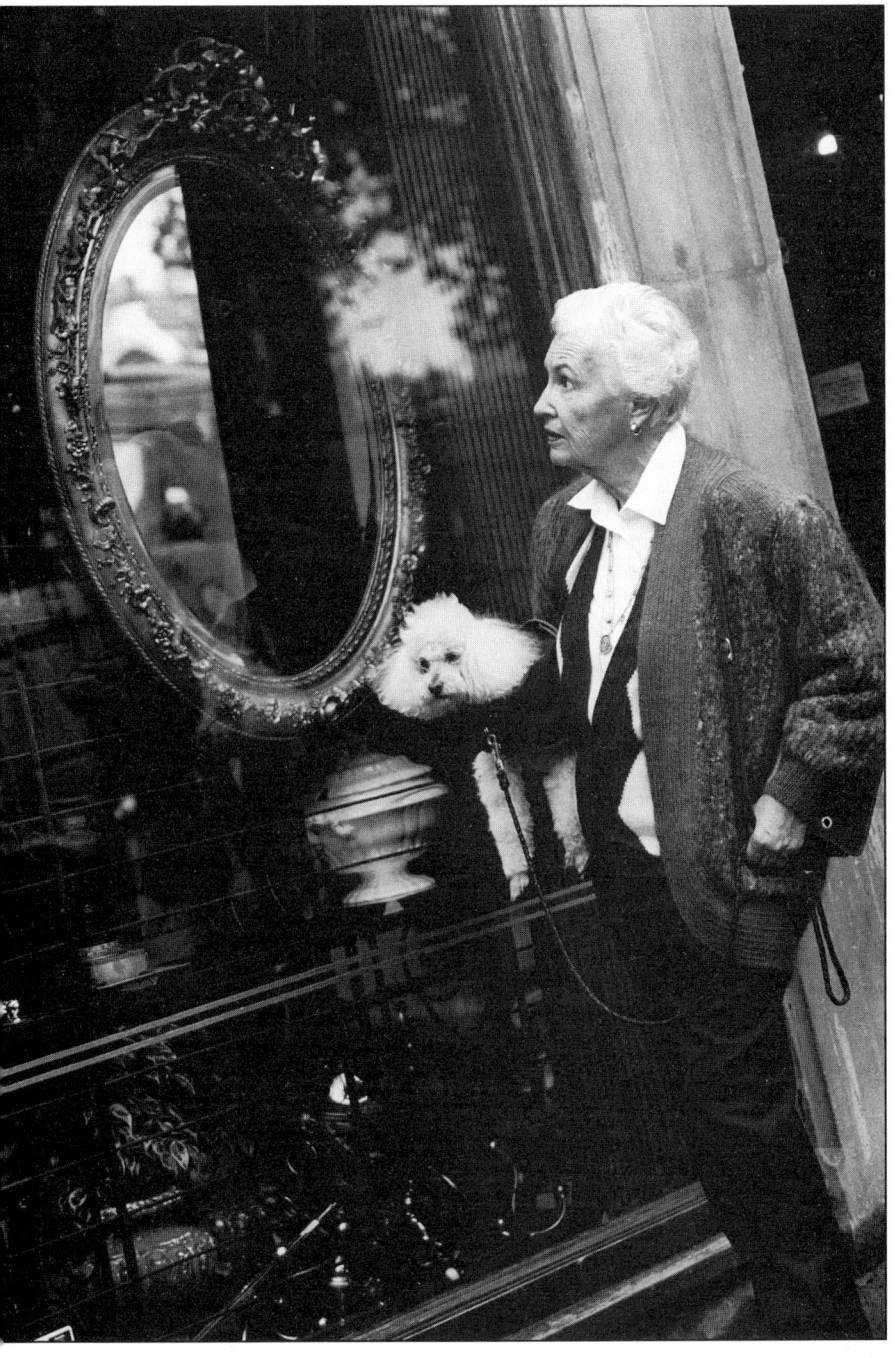

rather hear *"I know what I like, I enjoy this room, I welcome you to it and hope you enjoy it too."*

One of the cardinal rules in decorating is being unpredictable, sometimes. Mixing up the use of rooms can be very liberating. An oversized bedroom can be used half as sleeping quarters, half as entertaining space with the clever use of colours and arrangement of furniture to separate functions. A sofa, chair, small tables, some cushions on the floor, transform your wasted corner of bedroom into an intimate parlour for friends. An odd-angled hallway was transformed into a dining room by a woman who found the original dining room too small (she converted that into a study) for her refectory-style table. Pictures, plants, a wash of colour on the previously off-white walls, turned her hall into a unique and interesting "room".

Personal touches are elegant in any room. Piles of books, framed photographs, small boxes and jars, add a richness that is beguiling. Some other interesting things to add character and style to your elegant room might include:

- ◆ A terrarium (earthy and mysterious)
- ◆ A large wicker birdcage with bird (not a parrot)
- ◆ Framed collections of shells/buttons/fossils/pressed flowers
- ◆ Mirrors; judiciously used they open up and enlarge a room and can create a lovely effect at night with the right lighting
- ◆ Fans: large, brilliantly coloured paper fans in front of the fireplace make a focal point and are practical in that they hide the fireplace when it's not in use.

An elegant home is important to an elegant woman. It's an expression of her personality, her good taste on show, a pleasurable retreat from the world. If it's a pleasure to her, sweet on the eye, friendly, warm, and willingly returned to by herself, family and friends, she's got it right.

How to make your sitting room more elegant in ten minutes
Assuming you have the symmetrical, predictable arrangement of one three-piece suite, one television, one coffee-

Homestyle

table, and a lamp, arranged in a boxed, unstylish way, you can add a touch of elegance by:

◆ Removing the chair from the three-piece and replacing it with a wooden rocker or a chair in a complementary but different fabric

◆ Adding two huge vases of fresh flowers to the room; adds colour and perfume

◆ Piling books and magazines on the table to give the room a reason to come into it

◆ Taking the curtains down and putting up blinds or shutters; changes a room's personality completely

◆ Encasing the television set in a cabinet, even a second-hand, country auction piece will polish up beautifully. Take the back off for the electrical bits and bobs, close the doors on the TV, which vastly improves the room

◆ Installing a large, leafy potted tree – more life and foliage is soothing

◆ Plonking down lots of loose but lush fabric cushions around the room

◆ Taking down that print of Winchester Cathedral and putting up a good quality black-and-white *large* poster, elegantly framed, of 1930s café society.

12 ♦ *Workstyle*

Working women can be divided into two categories: those with jobs and those with careers. Women with jobs tend to be secretaries, clerks and sales staff; career women manage in business, are doctors, lawyers, teachers. Within these divisions, there are women working full-time, part-time, temporary, seasonally and job-sharing. But *all* working women find as they get older, that their place in the working scheme of things alters subtly, as does their attitude towards employment. Surprisingly, it's mostly good news. "*After twenty years working with male architects I became aware of a change in their attitude towards me. They had a great deal more respect and interest in my work and ideas. They'd decided I was here to stay because I was good and could no longer be dismissed as a pushy young woman, the female interloper. I was a fellow professional who had stature,*" a woman architect says. "*It shouldn't take half a working lifetime but it's still nice when it happens. I'm happier working now than at any other time in my life.*"

"**You do gain the respect of your peers,**" another woman says. "*Younger staff look up to you to sort out problems and management depends on you. They trust you now, it's as simple as that.*"

"*You gain a lot of common sense and confidence,*" says Peta Rogers, who's won and lost her share of jobs. "*Younger people panic when things go wrong, but a mature and experienced woman keeps her head and gets the job done. You may lose some of your looks when you get older, but you gain a lot of sense and experience which is far more valuable.*"

Workstyle

The process of gaining all this sense and experience is usually painful at the time. Kari-Ann Moller has particular sympathy for women when they start work, especially if they've been away from it for some time. *"You have to be tough to get along in the working world and being at home doesn't make for that toughness,"* she says. *"If you've been away for a few years you have to build it up again. There are bound to be a few weepies when you start back at work, but that's okay, that's part of it."*

When it comes to experiences to weep over, Peta Rogers has a complete collection. Any woman hesitating about stepping out in the workforce or considering a new job or position, harken. Looking back from the perspective of seventy-plus she can see how funny and character building her *faux pas* were, and what interesting dinner-party conversation they provide, but at the time she was shattered. Every woman who has felt suicidal at some ghastly error at work should take comfort from the confident, sensible, achieving Peta who went from the inept to the in-charge during her career. As you pore over the ads looking for another job, consider: *"One of the first jobs I had was packing in the basement of a big fashion house – nine a.m. to seven p.m. and for only one pound a week, so I was always hungry,"* Peta recalls. *"I used to persuade three of the saleswomen to buy buns from a nearby bakery because they were four for tuppence and I'd get to eat the left-over one, you see. One day I was packing up this gorgeous dress in layers of tissue paper and couldn't find my bun but just assumed I'd wolfed it down. The next day, a furious customer rang up; she'd unpacked her lovely dress to find sticky bun and icing all over it – I'd dropped it into the tissue packing of course. I got fired, but I was so thin and pale from working there, I got started in modelling."*

Being totally inexperienced, that career didn't get off to a roaring start either.

"I had plenty of crushing experiences in the beginning," Peta admits, *"I could write a book on doing it all the wrong way. I remember having to model a chiffon tea-gown to show it to buyers, and when I was putting it on, I discovered it was all but frontless! I was shocked and refused to part with my

vest and *I kept my hands folded across my chest when I walked on to the runway. The buyers were shouting 'let's see it', but I refused to lower my arms. Then one of them said, 'oh, no, she's got it on* backwards.' *That didn't do much for my modelling career I can tell you."*

Somehow from this inauspicious beginning, she salvaged enough ego, perseverance and experience to carry on and become head model at several of the top couture houses. She also worked occasionally with some of the top photographers of the era. From the legendary Norman Parkinson she picked up a certain amount of nonchalance in the face of on-the-job upset. *"Parks and I were shooting a* Vogue *feature in the underground in London; I had to get on and off a train at Piccadilly Circus at rush hour. Parks was sitting on a bench on the platform taking photos of me hopping on and off this train. It was very crowded and of course trains only stop a few minutes so I had to be quick. People must have thought I was a glamorously dressed mad woman, hopping on and off a dozen times so Parks could get his picture. 'What will I do if the doors shut before I can get off?' I asked him. Very coolly he replied, 'you'll go as far as Cockfosters, the train doesn't go any further.' That sort of unflappability has stayed with me."*

Confidence, calm, common sense – they are as valuable in the workplace as in the rest of life and mature women have them in abundance. In addition to growing more confident and comfortable with the responsibility and pressures of work, women, particularly career women, start to put their work life into perspective at this time. *"Since turning forty I've reassessed my career,"* a business woman says. *"I've worked so hard for so long now, I want a broader life. I want to open my life up. I've decided my life is more than just my job. It was for a long time and I'm still ambitious but I want to make room now for other things.*

"I've discovered that if you have no home life, no outside interests, no personal relationships, when things go wrong at work, life looks very black. I couldn't see it ten or even five years ago, but I can see it now."

One way or another the middle years for most working

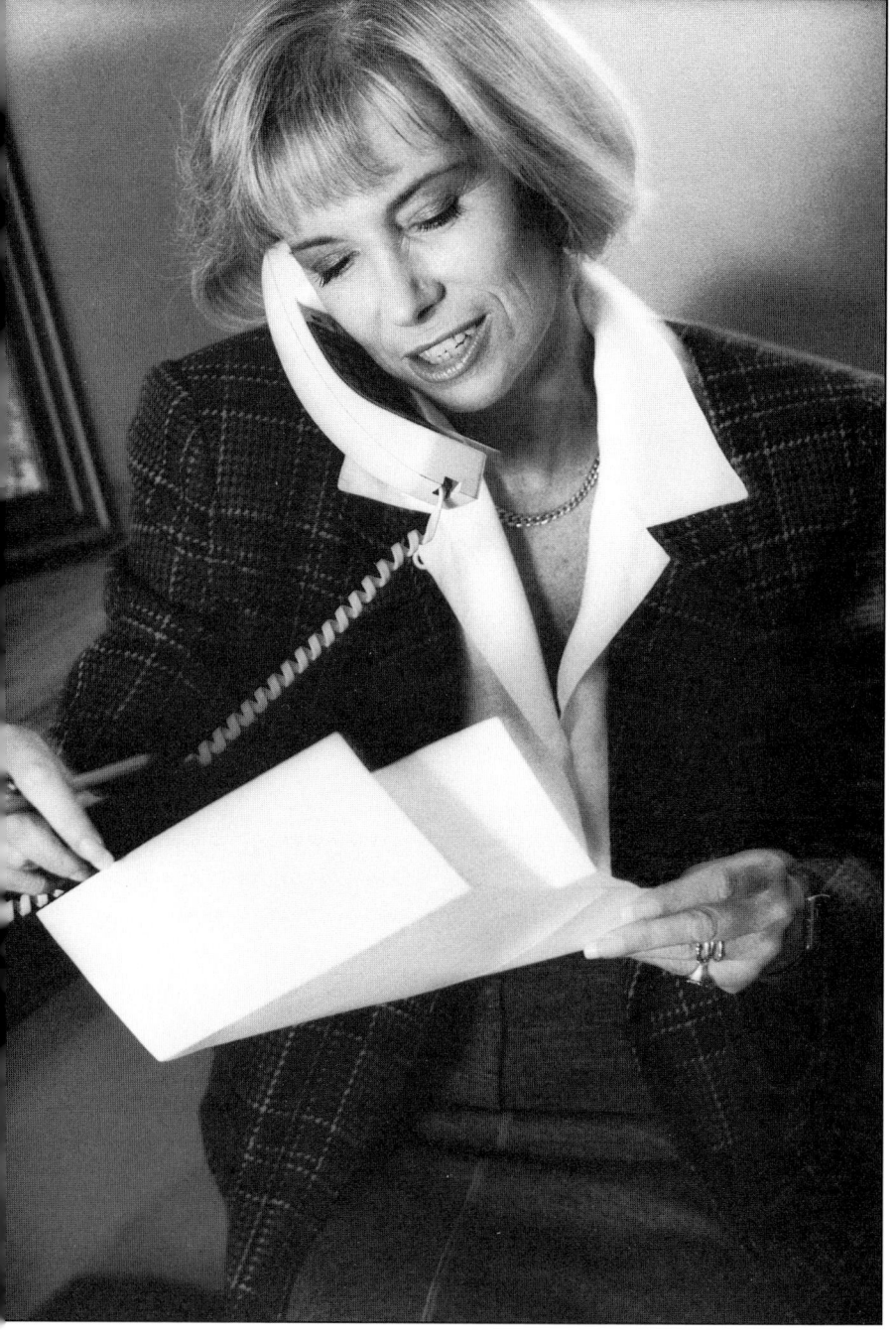

women are a time of decision and adjusting the balance. Many career women choose to go for broke and aim for the top; others are content with what they've achieved so far and decide to step off the treadmill and concentrate on building up a well-rounded life. Mature years can be the best for the get-ahead career woman, as many of the distractions and personal tugs of her twenties and thirties finally let go. Career women with young families are among the most distracted, living-on-the-edge, overtired people on earth. As they get older and their children get older and develop lives of their own, a great deal of their mental and emotional energy is suddenly freed up, to say nothing of the physical freedom in not having to rush home from work to do the evening chauffeuring shift – ballet, piano, Brownies and football practice. Most working mothers have the running of the household as their second full-time career so shedding it, its tiredness and divided mind, is truly liberating.

Mid-life is also the time of marital crisis, and some women find they are facing a divorce. Far from unsettling their careers, a recent American study showed that newly single women may flourish at work. A divorce gave a definite career boost, once the grieving was over, as women were freed of the responsibility for the relationship and were no longer the emotional anchor of another's life – all their effort and energy could be poured into their career. Whether you decide to slow down or pick up the career pace, the renaissance is a working watershed.

Any woman, high or low in any hierarchy, whether in a job or a career, full- or part-time, shares similar problems and faces some of the same difficulties.

Elegant working women carry on and through these difficulties with the same assured style they apply in their personal life and interests outside the office. A great deal of getting on in the working world depends on how well you interpret and act on the unspoken rules or hidden agenda; most women, by the time they've reached this age, have figured it out for themselves. But for those who have recently returned to work, or find themselves promoted to a new and more complex arena, or who, like Peta Rogers, find life

Workstyle

exceptionally full of banana peels to slip on when you least expect it, here are some guidelines to work by.

How to work successfully with men: As women get older they find many of the problems of antagonism and resentment they had with male peers, colleagues and bosses disappear as they gain in experience and stature. Unfair as it is, most women still find they have to prove they're right for the work, and it takes a long time before many men believe it. As accomplishments pile up over the years, it gradually sinks in, even into the most Neanderthal colleague, that your work is as important to you as his is to him, that you take your responsibility and position seriously and you never give less than your best. It hastens the acceptance process and helps men see you as a colleague and working partner and good manager if "professional" is your middle name:

◆ Never flirt. You're at work to work, not play. Topics of conversation that are best suited for the bar, provocative gestures and suggestive language, even in fun among colleagues you know well, may act against you.

◆ Dress to work. Anything too tight, too short or too revealing is too tasteless for work. You want your co-workers, men included, to notice your work, not your clothes. An elegant, understated dress sense sacrifices nothing of femininity but speaks volumes of strictly business.

◆ Don't take work personally. Women tend to take words and actions personally and to heart. Business men are familiar with the saying "today's enemy is tomorrow's ally". Women, if insulted and wounded, tend to pull up the drawbridge and declare an enemy for life. It isn't so in business. At a business studies group for trainee managers of both sexes, each member of the group strongly criticised the others' work and leadership skills as part of the programme. After the session broke up, all the women, miffed, feeling snubbed and hurt and let down by their colleagues even in this mock-up situation, went their separate ways, noses in the air. The men, sessions over, slapped each other on the back and went to lunch together. In business, it's not personal, just business, and women who can't roll with the punches, who let themselves be drawn in personally, won't survive happily.

◆ Don't talk with your hands. Many women have the annoying habit of pointing or even wagging their finger when making a point. There are few things more irritating to a man; it must remind him of an admonishing mother. If you watch two speakers at a seminar, one male, one female, you'll notice the male uses his whole, open hand to indicate something on the display or presentation. A woman uses her finger. When mother told you it was rude to point, she should have added it's bad for business too.

◆ Don't confide personal or intimate details of your private life to men at work, even colleagues you've known for a long time. Most men are uncomfortable with emotional revelations and they will use it against you.

◆ Don't feel you have to like everyone you work with. Women more than men are concerned with the emotional comfort of those around them. Admirable in most circumstances but not always workable at the office. You can hate someone with a passion but the professional in you has got to put it to one side and work beautifully in harness with him. You can know that a co-worker dislikes you, but it will never show in your work or public attitude when you're working together. That smoothly working grace under pressure is true elegance in the workplace.

How to dress for success: Of all the issues in the working world, this is the one that won't go away. Obviously, the first rule for dressing for anywhere, work, play, day or evening, is appropriateness. It's especially true at work. You can wear jeans and boots if you're the manager of a construction site. You can wear a leopardskin bra and red patent leather heels if you're a receptionist at an avant-garde recording company or art gallery. Or you can wear an elegantly cut suit and silk blouse if you're working in an investment house, bank, or any office where chic efficiency is needed. Having said that:

◆ Always dress for the job one higher than the one you've got. Senior management can't think of promoting

Workstyle

you if they don't see you in the role and they won't see you in the role if you're always kitted out like a junior typist.

◆ Always wear stockings or tights, never bare legs. It's more finished.

◆ Flat shoes or low heels, like court pumps, are better than stilettos unless you work in Soho.

◆ Suits are more versatile than dresses and two good suits and a variety of blouses make an easy mix and match wardrobe. They don't have to be sombre. There's no restriction on the use of colour; it's the line, shape and quality of the cut and style that counts. Cotton, linen, wool, silk, suede, are great fabrics for the office. Velour, denim, corduroy are not.

◆ Don't wear loud, flashy jewellery, especially earrings. Big is okay, but it's got to be quality and part of an overall "look".

◆ Don't carry a gigantic handbag, a briefcase plus small handbag is more elegant.

◆ Keep make-up and perfume subtle; hair looks more businesslike off the face. Wild, frizzy locks rarely make an elegant business look.

Speaking in public: Sooner or later you're likely to be called upon to make some sort of public speech at work. If you're a career woman in management this will be part of your job, whether addressing junior staff or making a presentation to senior management. Many companies provide training seminars for up-and-coming executives so they can learn and practise skills like public speaking and making effective presentations. Others throw them in the deep end and wait and see if they have the confidence and savvy to extract themselves. Most women of your age do. It's one of the advantages of being just that much older than a younger competitor. Any woman having to speak publicly should know there are two kinds of public speaking: off the cuff, and from notes. Off the cuff is for trained, nerveless, natural performers. The rest, about ninety-nine per cent of the speaking population, need a few notes. Small note-cards with memory-jogging key phrases may be all you need, not a prepared text which often

TOTAL ELEGANCE

sounds false and looks amateurish. Before you make your first speech:

◆ Get all the practice you can beforehand. Make your speech at home, for your husband, children, the window cleaner, the dog, Michael Buerk on the *Nine O'Clock News* . . .

◆ Take a deep breath before you begin to talk, to get some air in your lungs and resonance in your voice.

◆ Before you actually begin speaking, pause for a second to gather your thoughts and gather your audience's attention. Very effective stage trick, this.

◆ Speak slowly. Most nervous speakers rush through their words, so deliberately slow yourself down.

◆ Don't try to "make a speech". Talk to a roomful of colleagues in the same conversational and natural tone you'd use to talk to one of them at the tea wagon.

◆ Talk in everyday language (or the language of your profession), not in flowery, overelaborate phrases because you are "making a speech".

◆ If you hate your voice and speaking is increasingly part of your job, invest in voice lessons. You won't be alone. Most politicians and other public figures take voice instruction.

◆ Don't fidget. There's nothing that will obscure your message as much as your squirms, wriggles, hair-pulling and standing on one leg like a flamingo. If possible, get behind a podium to hide nervous body language.

◆ Always wear something absolutely comfortable, flattering and familiar. Don't wear something new you aren't used to. A management team at a large company were treated to the perplexing sight of a nervous woman speaker obviously missing her comfortable old suit which must have had a breast pocket in which she was used to putting a handkerchief, pens or note-cards or something, because throughout her talk she nervously patted her bosom from time to time, looking faintly surprised there wasn't a pocket there. No one remembered a thing she said. If it still feels like trial-by-ordeal, invest in a public speaking course, frequently offered in evening classes, by women's groups (often in conjunction with assertiveness training courses) or by management consultancies whose job it is to train people just like you to succeed in business.

Stereotypes: Stereotypes trip a lot of well-meaning women up. If your work situation changes – you may be promoted to a management position or you may find another career-track woman becomes your new boss – don't fall back on tired old stereotypes. Women bosses have enough trouble with unenlightened male colleagues without getting it from their female peers too. A stereotypical woman boss is always, according to her detractors, too soft to make decisions, too emotional to handle a crisis, too pushy and overbearing, incapable of making decisions quickly, uses sex to rise in the company and holds other women back. How often have you thought these things about other women? How often do you think colleagues have thought it about you? None of the stereotypes is any more true of a woman boss than a man, as any woman who has worked with sulking, dithering, disorganised, unreliable male bosses knows. *All* bosses, regardless of sex, fall into two categories: capable, visionary and fair, and incapable, blinkered and unjust. Sex is incidental.

How to deal with younger colleagues: Like the old saw about the policemen getting younger, it's true that women in their mid-forties onwards are seen as the older office generation by the bulk of rising young male and female staffers. Ageism is dying but it's not quite dead yet.

Peta Rogers remembers being recommended for a job on the assumption she was under forty. In actual fact she was forty-four, but the person promoting her didn't know it. Had senior management known, she wouldn't have been hired, she was told later, despite the fact they loved her work. Today she says that blatant discrimination is dying out. *"People of all ages talk, socialise and work together,"* she says. *"There isn't the segregation of older women there used to be."*

Perhaps not, but many older women view up-and-coming junior executives as threatening know-it-alls; in turn, the juniors regard the older, experienced doyennes as tough competition but essentially past it. But it only takes one big crisis to unlock all those years of experience, coolheadedness, nerve and verve to show the juniors where the confidence, ability and power lies. However, in the natural on-going progression of office life, it is likely that some of these younger women will rise and be your peers or successors one day, so it is much more elegant to be fair on all counts:

◆ Give them the benefit of your experience, advice and practical help if they ask for it; you can offer once, if you see someone really struggling, but you're not obliged to nanny anyone who's foolish enough to rebuff your help.

◆ If someone praises a junior's work, don't be jealous enough to disclaim it; you want good, strong, talented people to work with. It makes a more challenging and interesting working environment for everyone. When they screw up, as they eventually will, monumentally, as you did at twenty-five and thirty-five, be kind. A sneer is *the* most inelegant thing to wear in the office.

Sexual harassment at work: Older women are not immune from this; the stereotype (again) of a twenty-year-old secretary being chased around a desk, is only one type of harassment. Older women, particularly those in management positions, find the real harassment starts here. They're often the only one or one of a few women at business meetings or conferences. Their work includes business lunches and dinners, situations that can easily waver over into the social arena. They occasionally travel out of town, sometimes with male co-workers. The scene is set for potential harassment but it doesn't have to happen. Your colleagues and senior management should know you well enough at this stage to respect your work and your self, in or out of the office, and treat you as a talented and trusted colleague, not as an eligible woman at dinner. Unfortunately there may be one who gets carried away with an expense account lunch. Most women at your age have long decided how to handle these sticky situations and are adept at extricating themselves from them. For those of you who are new to it, or never got the hang of it, or have been lucky enough not to be confronted with it, there are a few protective ground rules, all self-evident:

◆ For business lunches and dinners, the rules of business, not social dressing, apply. No plunging necklines or short

Workstyle

skirts; you want an elegant conservative look because no matter how luxurious or exotic the setting, it's still part of the business day.

◆ Don't address senior partners in a familiar way just because you're out of the office confines, and don't let anyone address you differently than they do in the office. If you're Mrs Smith at the office, you're Mrs Smith around the conference table, if it's always been "Jane", fine – "honey" or "dear" is never fine.

◆ Drink sparingly. Mineral water is more than acceptable these days at any function. If you are drinking alcohol, remember that excitement, the tiredness of business travelling and the natural stress of the circumstances make a drink especially potent and cut back.

◆ If a man comes on aggressively, don't panic – cut him short right away, and move away if you can – *"I'm here on business, Mr Jones, excuse me"*. You don't want a scene but you don't want to feel under attack either. If you're sitting next to someone and can't move, engage your neighbour in conversation and give your pursuer the chance to join in. At future groupings arrange to enter, sit with and leave with another woman at the meeting or a male colleague you know and can depend on.

Particularly tough and confident and well-practised women find their own ways around sexual harassment. One woman who refused her boss's advances found he tried to pressure her with one-upmanship. *"If you won't, I'll say you did,"* he threatened. *"If you say you did,"* she countered, *"I'll say you couldn't."* He retreated. You can handle it any way that's comfortable to you. The more dignified the better, but if you have to take the gloves off, don't hesitate.

Occasionally harassment goes beyond the irritating, unpleasant and embarrassing, and mushrooms out of manageable proportions. No woman need suffer. If, after confronting your harasser you get no assurance he'll stop, go to your immediate superior and make a formal complaint. But go in armed with specifics not generalities: list, on paper, dates and times and details of incidents, physical and verbal. If you're a member of a union, there is likely to be an employee committee that deals specifically with harassment. Government offices, local councils and universities may have a special committee or ombudsman who deals with such complaints. If your immediate superior refuses to take notice, you're justified in going over his or her head. But the most vital thing to remember is to approach the problem rationally and constructively, and present yourself as an intelligent, collected and capable professional, not an emotional, overwrought virago, however you may feel inside.

Maintaining an elegant workstyle spills over from your general elegant attitudes to life. The confidence to handle the job, assurance to take on bigger challenges if you want them, the maturity to deal with all kinds of people and personalities, and do it with good manners and style, is all part of an elegant spirit in the workplace. All work is about service, whether you're serving literally in a restaurant or a shop, or whether you're a doctor providing a medical service, or a politician providing a government service. Good service is about good manners, something the elegant woman has in abundance. Using your talents to the full is elegant; providing that extra little bit of service, unasked, is elegant too. A sense of responsibility, pride in your work, taking yourself and your job seriously and being dedicated to getting it right and giving your best, is very elegant. Laziness, shirking responsibility, blaming others when things go wrong, is not.

◆ ◆ ◆

A major blow to many women in middle-age is redundancy – all of a sudden after years in a good position, the carpet is pulled out from under you, in the biggest career crunch of all. Sometimes it's a slew of front-line workers that go, sometimes a company purges middle management as the most likely layer of padding to thin out. Occasionally a woman finds losing her job opens new doors and is the best career thing to happen in a long time. *"It forced me to take a risk I never would have taken,"* says a woman who was let go after nineteen years in fashion retailing. She wept for a week, then marshalled her energy and skills and started a fashion consultancy, advising businesswomen on wardrobes, choosing, shopping, creating business images. *"I wouldn't go back to*

Workstyle

working for anyone else now," she says. *"I've taken a lifetime of retailing experience and am putting it to work for myself. I sink or swim by myself. It's a bit frightening, but it's a very powerful feeling too. I wouldn't trade it in."*

But losing a job, any job, is for most a painful shock, and the first forty-eight hours a walking nightmare. There's little consolation in the fact you're not alone, that there are thousands who have lost their jobs too. There's some comfort when you put it into perspective: your confidence lets you see that although you are temporarily jobless, you are not worthless, talentless or powerless. There's no shame in losing a job, so:

♦ Don't hide the fact you're out of work, and don't stop thinking of yourself as employable. Many women go into a blue funk, sleeping late, driven by depression and anxiety. Take twenty-four hours to go mad if you must, then get on with getting another job. Now is the time to start calling in all those IOUs of business acquaintances for introductions, and gossip about new job openings. Get a good CV (see page 142) together and start calling people calmly and methodically. Lunch with still-working contacts, keep in touch with former colleagues, keep up subscriptions to professional journals: all are sources of employment.

♦ Most companies are hurt by redundancies as much as the people laid off. They don't enjoy it and it's usually caused by market forces beyond their control. So, when you're lunching with colleagues, don't badmouth the company or vent your spleen to the opposition. That really is inelegant.

♦ Don't hide your feelings of anger, fear, disappointment and hurt from your family and close friends. Losing a job is traumatic. You'd have to be superhuman not to reel a little from the shock of it. Don't deny yourself your best sources of comfort, support and good humour when you need them most.

Elegant women, at home or work, know that taking from loved ones when you need it is as important as giving when they need you.

TOTAL ELEGANCE

Three elegant things to do at work
1   Buy a stressed-out colleague some fresh flowers for her desk.
2   Volunteer to switch shifts with a co-worker desperate to get away to a sick child, new date, family reunion.
3   Stay late or take home some extra work because your new boss is pressed to the limit and in need of a steadying hand on the tiller.

Three inelegant things to do at work
1   Gossip unremittingly about colleagues.
2   Indulge in a little petty theft because the company will never miss a bit of paper, some pens, typewriter cartridges, envelopes or magazines from the reception desk.
3   Deliberately make life difficult for a new woman boss because you prefer working for a man.

13 ♦ *Lifestyle*

Life's patterns change as a woman enters her renaissance years. Priorities shift, old responsibilities fall away, new interests absorb her energy.

For women with children, the lifestyle of the past twenty years drops away as children find their own path in the world, away from home, and new interests fill the vacuum. Family life has such a different rhythm from the life of a couple or single woman. Just as the arrival of a child makes a hitherto unguessed-at impact in the early years, so their leaving the nest makes an equally unsettling and unexpected impression. This time around though, instead of giving up or putting aside something of herself in a willing sacrifice to her children, a woman can reclaim her self and her time.

"When the children were growing up, everything was for them, as it should be," recalls Frances Meachem. *"But now I have a freedom I haven't had since they were born. Life revolved around them for years as it does with most parents. You do an awful lot that goes unthanked at the time. Not that you expect thanks and praise all the time, but you do give a lot of yourself. Even if you wouldn't have it any other way, it doesn't make it easy. You give them the best you can for as long as you can, but then it's time to take charge of your own life again. You spend so much time wrapped up in your children that it's often quite difficult when they become adults, but then no transition is easy."*

Wanting to let them go, but keeping the door open, treating them one moment like children because they act like it, the next like adults which in terms of years they are . . . *"you have to be hard eventually and say 'stand on your own',"*

Frances Meachem says. "Encourage them to stand on their own two feet but they have to know you're there if they really need you, that they can come back any time. It's difficult for them and very stressful for a mother, seeing them as adults, but feeling *they're still your children.*"

Pat Knight, whose son is now at university, says the relationship between only children and parents has its own pitfalls. "It's tricky with an only child because the relationship can become so intense," she says. "It's one to one all the time with no siblings to dilute it. They become very sensitive to atmosphere. You risk smothering rather than mothering but I've been wary of that and tried to back off and let him make his own decisions and own mistakes as he's got older. Only children can become the repository of their parents' anxieties and expectations, and even end up feeling more responsible for their parents than they should, which isn't fair. One has to juggle their needs and space with one's own needs and space."

It's difficult for a woman to keep silent while watching her children make painful and foolish mistakes. The urge to interfere, to jump in and protect them, to sort out their messes, is ingrained after years of child raising. "I had to almost physically restrain myself from rushing to their aid," one honest empty-nester says. "For a year or two after they left home, they'd call every time a crisis hit, at home, work, with friends, or when they couldn't figure out how things worked in the system out there. But I realised that they only came running when things were difficult or aggravating, not when all was sweetness and light. I wasn't sharing their life, as I kept telling myself I was, I was just digging them out of their bad times. I felt then I had to let them cope with the disasters as well as the pleasures of independence. When my daughter locked herself out of her flat and called for help, I said don't come round, sort it out yourself. She eventually did what any adult would do – call a locksmith. It was a much better solution for her, if rather expensive, than coming round to sleep here and waiting till her flatmate got back into town next day with another key."

But the practical problems seem like nothing compared to

Lifestyle

the emotional ones. Says one woman watching her daughter in the throes of a miserable love affair: *"We told her from the beginning that the boy was hopeless and would make her miserable but she wouldn't listen. I remember feeling like that about some ghastly man when I was her age. The only way, sadly, to develop good judgement about people, is trial and error, as hurtful as it may be. I kept quiet, she got her heart broken – as I did and probably my mother and grandmother did too, but she'll mend: the rest of us did."*

Frances Meachem agrees *"you can't lead their lives for them. You have such experience at this age and you can see the mistakes they're making and long to spare them. But getting hurt is part of the growing-up process; they have to be allowed to make their own mistakes and suffer for them."*

But sympathetic and generous by nature, elegant parents stand by, if not to catch their sons and daughters before they fall, at least to pick them up and dust them off and offer an empathetic shoulder to cry on. It's always difficult to stand this far back from people you love, but it's easier if, in addition to the adjustment of letting go, you also grab something for yourself elsewhere. *"This is a great age to start new interests and projects,"* Frances Meachem says. *"I'm a great believer in revamping a lifestyle from time to time. Women must never say it's too late, they can't start anything new now. I was complaining about just that to a friend, saying I was too old to do something or other, and he said 'well how old will you be if you* don't *do it?' It's a great point. It isn't age that stops you doing anything, it's attitude."*

Tania Mallet agrees. *"Reaching this middle stage of life happens very quickly, rather like the end of term. Suddenly it's just there and you can put your self-interest first after years of looking after others. This can be a really wonderful age. Women shouldn't waste time mourning their youth. At this age you've still got looks plus lots of experience and confidence, and more freedom to fashion a lifestyle that suits you. Life seems much more on your terms."* Says Pat Knight, *"At this time of life, women need to do things for themselves for sheer pleasure and ego and enjoyment. After years of looking after children or slaving at a career, or both, you reach a point where you can be a bit selfish, and live for yourself.''*

An "elegant lifestyle" doesn't mean Cowes, Henley and Ascot and swanning around town buying hats. It does mean living your life to the full, honestly, richly, giving out as well as taking the best, setting and pursuing your own standards.

It means branching out into long neglected personal pursuits, broadening and enriching your life. An elegant lifestyle also encompasses reaching out to people beyond the comfortable circle of family and friends. Many women take up volunteer or charity work, putting generous and empathetic qualities to practical use. *"When you're young, you get on with life and make your mark,"* says a recent recruit to volunteer work. *"But at this time of life you look around and see how truly fortunate you are. It's time to put something back, reach out; you can afford to do it now."*

In their own circle, women may find this life-stage heralds more entertaining, one area where an elegant woman should be a confident success. Entertaining fulfils so many needs: it's social, bringing life, stimulation, conversation and new people into a woman's home; it's a source of warmth and stability as old friends continue to stay close; it's good for her ego and feelings of value to see people enjoying her home and her company. Unfortunately, just the word "entertaining" is enough to send some women scurrying for cover, especially those whose recent memories of parties over the last few years are all about jelly and crisps trodden into the carpet or beer cans and a broken stereo from a teenage rave-up, or the annual pre-Christmas affair which, after the shopping, cooking, wrapping and general frenetic build-up to the season, she's too exhausted to enjoy. You can put all that behind you now and relax – part of the new lifestyle is that entertaining on any scale becomes a pleasure. Elegant entertaining is based on a simple premise that it has nothing to do with the expense or elaborate presentation of food and drink. It rests simply on the comfort and enjoyment of guests. If you spend hours and a sultan's fortune preparing intricate dishes, served on priceless china, set in an immaculate room and your guests feel so intimidated they can hardly swallow, it was not an elegant

Lifestyle

evening. If you hand around baskets and platters of sandwiches while you sit on cushions in front of the fire and everyone is thoroughly relaxed and happy, elegance pervades the room.

A well-planned and well-executed dinner party is within the grasp of every woman, especially now she's old enough to enjoy it. *"I used to dread sitting between two strangers at dinner when I was younger,"* says Tania Mallet, *"I had no store of information, no titbits, no fount of knowledge to carry on conversations. It's only as you get older that you acquire, through living, all kinds of small talk and bits and pieces that will carry you through a conversation easily. The confidence it gives! Dinner parties aren't for the young!"*

When Isabella Beeton published her famous book on household management in the 1860s, she separated dining experiences into "elaborate" and "elegant". The message hasn't changed: simple and well-prepared dinners can be far more elegant and fun than complicated, laborious affairs. In her culinary bible, Mrs Beeton advises: *"It is almost impossible to appear utterly unconcerned when one is harassed by petty cares and a thoroughly good hostess is one who is able herself to enjoy, without anxiety, the dinner she is giving to her friends."* Her voice carries down to us more than a century later and we are grateful for the excellent advice which still stands.

To simplify it further, here is a brief, and not Beetonesque (her *Household Management* ran to 1,644 pages), guide to entertaining, broken down to essentials of who, what, when, where, how.

Who: Party lists do change over the years. *"I never liked entertaining people for the sake of it, because you 'owe' them,"* says Frances Meachem. *"We had enormous parties when we lived in the country, sometimes one hundred people. I asked everyone because I wanted to be asked everywhere back. When you're younger you can't bear to miss out on anything, but I think women at this age should stop doing this. You deserve to spend your time with people you really like, whose company lifts you. The days of duty entertaining* *are over. Friends are so important, I selfishly spend all possible time with them."*

"*I don't like dinner parties to be predictable, formal affairs,*" says Kari-Ann Moller, "*so I like to have lots of different types of people, all professions, mixed up together. I like it to be a little intriguing and for the mix to create an element of mystery — mystery is very elegant to me.*" Children at Pat Knight's parties are made part of it by being allowed to hand the food around before dinner. "*It breaks the ice for everyone and gets everyone involved.*" Sandra Paul says she was advised to always have "*a shouter*" at the party, someone with no inhibitions, an extrovert, a good talker, to get things going. She and her husband double-check — "*have we got a good shouter?*" when drawing up guest lists.

What: A dinner party is one of the most elegant forms of entertaining at home. However, it does have alarming overtones of Edwardian grandeur for some women. Such formality! Such etiquette! Such expense! Such nonsense! A dinner party can be as grand as a family wedding feast or as simple as a summer buffet for two or three close couples. It is neither as daunting nor as difficult as women imagine — the key is to create a party in your own style, not try and ape something showy that makes you uncomfortable and feels false. "*We like to have a formal sit-down dinner because it suits our friends,*" says Sandra Paul, "*but there are no hard and fast rules.*" "*We've given up sit-down affairs unless there are a lot of older members of the family,*" says another great entertainer. "*Buffets free people up, they force them to get up and move around and make small talk while they're helping themselves to food; we have lots of chairs and several small tables around our largest room and people manage with that. A lot of them end up sitting on the floor even in their fanciest clothes but it doesn't seem to matter. It makes for a very lively party. You can't not talk to someone when you're sharing an ottoman.*"

When: The rule used to always be Saturday night for dinner parties, a veteran hostess recalls, but there's less rigidity now and people have dinners any night of the week. "*I love it — it gets rid of that false separation between week and weekend.*"

Lifestyle

But, adds another, weekends should be sacrosanct for friends if you're a woman who has to give, or go to, a lot of business dinners in the week, although sometimes the two do cross over. Winter is best for me for dinner parties, Kari-Ann Moller says. *"In the summer our lives are given over to cricket."*

Summer is *the* best time for dinners because you can turn the whole thing into a picnic and eat alfresco in the garden, insists another woman. You must see your friends as much as possible, says one woman, but real stops-out dinner parties are for special occasions. I couldn't agree with that, a third woman counters, some of the loveliest dinners I've been to have been last-minute things that were pulled together by the warmth of the hostess and the good humour and appreciation of her guests. Obviously the when of giving a party takes care of itself – whenever you feel like giving one is a great time. Some parties become mini-institutions in a social circle – the Jones' bonfire night buffet, the Smiths' New Year's Day goose dinner, the Greens' mid-summer barbeque – they become as much a part of the social calendar as Christmas or birthdays. And when do all these parties end? *"Great parties are the ones that go on for ever,"* Kari-Ann Moller says. *"It's wonderful giving a party that nobody wants to leave."*

Where: A great deal of business entertaining is not done at home at all, but in restaurants, a very good thing as far as most women are concerned. Producing a meal under scrutiny from bosses, colleagues and an anxious partner rattles even the most proficient hostess.

If you must go this route, have it catered for if you can (and most women in a position to do business entertaining can afford a caterer) and rent the works: tablecloths, glasses, china; hire a florist. It's amazing how liberating other people's possessions are, and it enforces the difference between a party for business and one for pleasure. When you have business contacts or acquaintances to dinner, it's not just the food and setting that's under scrutiny. The house and its inhabitants have to measure up. Although, again, the women who are entertaining on this scale will have the perfect backdrop already, it's not a bad idea to let the children sleep over at granny's or a friend's to avoid an eight-year-old blurting out *"so you're the incompetent pillock who keeps Mum late every Friday night"*, or something similar. Board the cat and dog too, in case your boss is allergic. *"My experience has been that most business entertaining is done in restaurants, thankfully,"* Sandra Paul says. *"It's easier on everyone, including the boss."*

Although most dinner parties are indoor affairs, summer brings the barbecues out. They too require some thought and planning for your guests' comfort. True, you can dispense with cloth napkins and use paper ones, but you must have decent outdoor furniture. You can't really eat spareribs perched on the edge of a stone urn. Barbecues are traditionally rained out too, so if you're planning a sylvan dinner you must have either (a) a marquee for sudden wet weather or (b) a room set up inside if the guests have to take cover.

How: Over the years many women will have developed traditionally successful methods of entertaining; others will have just reached a stage where they feel they can give the kind of parties they like. *"For years parties have meant chips and fish fingers for our children's school chums. One of the first things I did when they got into their teens was take a cookery course and now I love having dinner parties. It was like discovering civilisation again,"* is how one woman put it.

Not everyone has the time, or in truth the interest, to concoct wondrous, perfectly executed dishes. But any woman can learn to make two or three decent things and always serve them. Good quality food properly cooked is all that's necessary and every woman is capable of that much. Most women have one or two steadfast rules. Sandra Paul avoids anything that needs carving, so might have a casserole or breast of duck. And for dessert, *"I love making ice creams so we usually have that with biscuits. People always eat cheese if it's put out. And you must serve real coffee, never instant, that is important."*

Some women are victims of their own success. Pat Knight makes treacle tart for a certain friend every time he comes to dinner. *"He loves it and he always knows he's going to get it,"* she smiles. *"It's a pleasure to make it for him because he enjoys it. I think doing special things for friends, showing you care, is very elegant."* It's true how well you treat your guests and how much trouble you take is a measure of how important they are, and how much you care for them. You don't eat the food when being entertained for nutritional value, but to be part of a gathering. Food fashions – pesto, sun-dried tomatoes, braised endive, cold fruit soups – come and go but manners, thoughtfulness and effort never go out of style.

"I do think that even though things are more relaxed than they once were, you do have to push the boat out a bit," Sandra Paul says. *"I don't take it too far down the line but good food and flowers are important."* Pat Knight agrees. *"I always have beautiful flowers in the house, they make such a difference to the atmosphere. And I do try and please guests. The treacle tart was one thing. I have a girlfriend who loves Freesias so I make sure I have them on the table when she's there. Looking after people and making them feel wanted is part of elegant entertaining. I like to cook so I go to some lengths to make sure the food is right – it's another way of showing people they're worth the effort."*

Kari-Ann Moller takes entertaining literally one step further than the food. *"I love to actually have some live entertainment,"* she says. *"I've had musicians and a storyteller. It creates a time when guests can sit and be amused and absorb the atmosphere. It breaks the ice. It takes people's minds off themselves and they really start mixing and relaxing together – you never know what you may be starting."*

Although most women, through habit, concentrate on the entertainment and food and let a husband or partner worry about the wine, every woman should know enough about wine to pick out something decent to go with what she is preparing. The number one rule is not to be intimidated by the deliberately confusing hype and hysteria that surrounds wine. Like everything else, wine is a matter of taste, although it's a good bet the ten-pounds bottle is going to be more palatable to most drinkers than the two-pounds one. But, if you like Bull's Blood and are serving a hearty goulash and have the dash to carry it off, go ahead. Please though, one small concession to convention: at least get a bottle with a cork in it, not a screw cap. Otherwise stick to mineral water. Other rules can be tossed overboard though: the old guideline about white wine with chicken and fish, red with red meat, is meaningless. It makes better gastronomic sense to match the wine with the type of food you are serving. For example, a plain roast deserves a good quality wine which won't overpower it, but a heavy Italian or some spicy, rich dish will taste just as good with a coarser, full-bodied wine. The shelves are crammed with so many possibilities the names blur before the eyes: Soave, Spätlese, Chianti, Vinho Verde, Frascati, Valpolicella – maybe *he'd* better choose the wine after all. Take heart though – generally speaking, it's pretty difficult to find a completely undrinkable Italian red or German white. Sweetness and dryness is such a personal taste, but in buying for a crowd, err on the side of dryness. Nothing's worse than sipping a wine that fills your mouth with flowery perfume. Supermarkets often have pamphlets or booklets available on choosing wine and sometimes feature a "wine of the week" which will at least be drinkable. The weekend supplements of most national newspapers and many women's and lifestyle magazines run regular wine features so you can top up your expertise.

Other than trusted friends' recommendations, finding wines you enjoy is a matter of taste. You can spend a pleasant few weeks uncorking several medium-price wines and trying them out, and drawing up a chart of the especially nice ones. It's not an indulgence, it's social investment. Oh do go on, uncork that one too.

As the party hour approaches, inexperienced hostesses often suffer an attack of stage fright. The time to go mad and have hysterics is before your guests arrive. Once the doorbell rings, it's time to stop labouring and let the evening happen, which is why it's so important to prepare something manageable and not a gargantuan, unwieldy spread. Don't be overambitious unless you're an experienced cook and hostess. Nothing is more stressful to guests than the suspicion their hostess is agonising in the kitchen, fussing with a hundred little finishing touches on a dinner that won't come together.

Lifestyle

It's also unfair to try out extreme dishes on guests, however much you love to shock your own tastebuds. Give them at least an option to seaweed pie, braised mole and garlic ice cream, although the last is reputed to be delicious. If your one and only dish is a strong one – hot curry for example – it is a mark of consideration and thoughtfulness to check with guests before the dinner to make sure they can all eat the food. Making your guests uneasy is the soul of inelegance, and there really is no excuse for the appalling bad manners that turn some dinner party circuits into a social battlefield of one-upmanship.

The tone of a dinner party is immediately set by the table, and as in clothing, attitude and behaviour, elegant simplicity wins out over fussy extremes. Although all party-givers have to make an effort, things are a lot simpler than in Mrs Beeton's day when party napkins were expected to be folded into elaborate shapes – the mitre, the rose, Cinderella's slipper, the Neapolitan, among others – and where the menu for one meal included soup, lobster, veal, duck, cheese soufflé, vegetables, apricot bouchées and coffee custard, all with the necessary cutlery. And the table centrepiece was flowers, ferns and small trees!

Every table benefits from some delicate decoration, usually flowers or candles or combinations of the two. Sticking a big vase of flowers dead centre is not much help at all. Table flowers need to be in a low, light and feathery arrangement so that dinner guests can see over or through them. There's nothing worse than trying to talk over a stiff, tall bunch of blooms that obscures faces opposite. The same consideration applies to candles, where a candelabra-type arrangement blocks both views and conversations. Feeling hemmed in isn't elegant, so don't overload the table with too much decorative art. A frequent party-goer recalls going to a Christmas dinner at the home of a well-known hostess who had laden her table with miniature Christmas trees, wrapped boxes, ribbons, candles and scattered pine-cones and baubles, so the effect was of eating in a chaotic department store display window. *"I held my elbows in the whole night,"* she says, *"afraid to knock something over."*

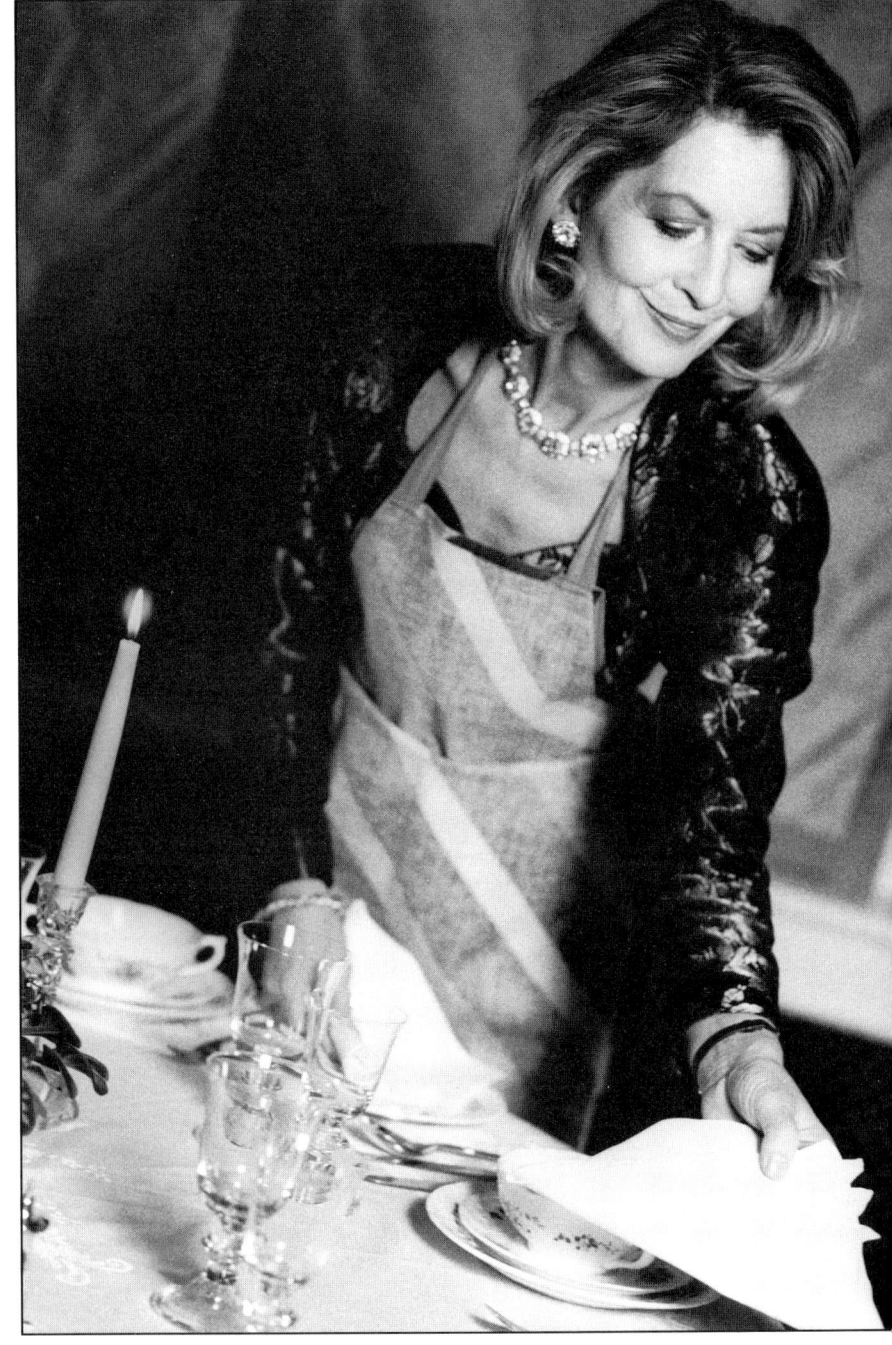

Lifestyle

Table décor doesn't have to be complicated to be elegant. You may use a cloth but if the table is lovely and a feature in itself, you'll want to show off the wood and just use place settings. Centrepieces can be constructed around the seasons, if you're looking for a theme: small fresh flowers and buds in spring, flowers and shells in summer, autumn leaves, berries and Michaelmas daisies in the autumn, pine branches and a few white sprays in winter.

Setting out the implements comes naturally to most hostesses. Forks on the left, spoons and knives on the right, with the blade edge of the knife towards the plate. The fork or knife to be used first placed farthest from the plate, so implements are used from the outer edge in. Bread and butter plates on the left. Wine glasses and coffee cups to the upper right. Serving spoons and forks to the right of their dishes. Left, right, left, right, maybe a buffet would be more comfortable? If you think your guests can manage on their laps it's a great idea, but lock up the dog so they can eat in peace.

Elegant women do not get in a flap when things go wrong, as they invariably do. Any upsets, spills or incipient scenes have to be carried off with aplomb on your part and visible kindness to the transgressor.

Sandra Paul's two best examples of coolheaded elegance in the face of disaster
1 *"Someone dropped a solid glass salad bowl on a glass table-top and broke both, plus some glasses on the table. Everyone, culprit and hostess remained very calm and matter-of-fact, as though shattered glass and splattered food were an everyday occurrence."*
2 *"Someone else had the caterers in for a big occasion, and a waiter slipped with the joint and the beef went flying off the platter on to the floor. The hostess calmly said 'Never mind, just bring in the other beef.' The waiter took the hint, retrieved the fallen beef and exited, returning with a joint on the platter. Of course it was the same joint, there was no other, but he'd picked up his cue from the hostess – and what presence of mind on her part!"*

TOTAL ELEGANCE

The absolutely most excruciating thing ever to happen at dinner
From an anonymous contributor: *"The fellow sitting across from me at this very formal and beautiful affair was flirting like mad with the woman next to him and obviously making progress. In an effort to impress her, he reached his hand into the centrepiece to pull out a flower to give to her, but in doing so he tugged the whole vase over, and water came spilling out, all over the table, over the edge into people's laps – gorgeous evening dresses and dinner suits; water and flowers were everywhere. Of course he was mortified; she looked like she'd turned to stone; drinks were spilled as people stood up too quickly to avoid the water – the entire table was ruined. I daresay his career was too."* Now, knowing that, you can forget about things going wrong at your dinner party, relax and enjoy it.

Three awful things to do at an elegant dinner
Refer to your napkin as a "serviette".
Cut your bread roll with a knife instead of breaking or tearing it.
Say, gosh I didn't know Bird's Eye did a smoked fish flan.

A good start and a great finish
Pat Knight's Kipper Pâté
Two kippers
Fromage frais   Cayenne pepper
Sea salt, black pepper
One tablespoon natural yoghurt
Poach or grill kippers. Remove skin and bones. Put all ingredients in a liquidiser and blend until smooth. Serve with toast or spread on to the hollows of celery sticks or chunks of wholemeal bread.

Sandra Paul's Home-made Ice Cream
Three large eggs
Three ounces of caster sugar
Three-quarters of a pint of double cream
Cook's choice of flavourings: chocolate, coffee granules, brandy, fruit, etc.
Separate eggs. Beat sugar with the egg yolks until pale. Add the cream and egg whites, beat, add assorted flavourings of your choice – "very strong melted marmalade is delicious" – and freeze.

14 ♦ *Menstyle*

An elegant woman's best accessory is an elegant man. If she's lucky she's already living with one. If she's determined, she may encourage the man she's got towards elegance, or go looking for a new one.

After all the desire and effort to be at your finest, it's back to earth with a jolt if your partner has taken a less becoming and inspiring path to middle life. Happily matched couples mature together, their basic good taste and similar interests ripening in unison. She continues to be an assured, well-groomed accomplished woman, and he never loses the style and flair that made him so attractive in the early years. Like her, he too explores new interests and develops a touch of the New Man mentality in his contributions to home and family care. He is good-humoured and generous, outgoing and full of interest in life, and always ready to learn or try anything new that interests him. His early style hasn't deserted him any more than yours has.

Other not-so-wonderfully paired couples wake up in mid-life to find they are poles apart. A great deal of the adventuring spirit is taken out of life by the realities and responsibilities of the hard-driving career and family years. Although you may arrive at mid-life bursting with energy and enthusiasm to go on to new things, he may be totally uninterested. He may have abandoned all efforts to keep up-to-date and be willing to sink into an undemanding and unattractive premature old age. It can be disheartening for a woman who feels the best part of her life is just beginning to be with a man who considers the best is behind them both. There's only so much holding back and denying yourself you can cope with, so many social events you go to alone, so many invitations you turn down, so many parties you don't give, before the rot of resentment sets in.

What this man needs is a woman who makes him confront the second, best, part of his life and enjoy it with her. Women, says Pat Knight, greatly fear the loss of physical attractiveness as they get older and fear losing the man in their life. This usually spurs them on to make the best effort with themselves, partly for their own pride, and partly to hang on to what they love. Men too must have some of that same fear and should have the same motivation to keep themselves in great shape and attitude. The defeatist who won't acknowledge this shouldn't be allowed to get away with giving up, for his own sake. Everyone wants to be admired and desired, no matter how out of the habit they've got. Your man really would rather be fit and trim and attractive than paying the physical price of too many business lunches and inactivity. Older men have a wealth of advantages. They are experienced, sophisticated and knowledgeable in the ways of the world, they are usually financially more secure than in their youth, they are sexually experienced and know enough about women to enjoy them and value their company rather than feel threatened or puzzled by them as younger men do. Men should feel as wonderful about reaching the middle of their life as women. But changing an old crocodile into an elegant man is uphill work for even the most determined woman.

If you have a man worth salvaging, an indirect approach rather than direct attack gets better results. Men's egos are eggshell. Tell him he's overweight, drinks and smokes too much and is a recluse, and you're lucky to get a grunt in response before he turns up the television. Invite him to go for a walk with you, prepare fresh, healthy meals with no fried rubbish and creamy desserts, and you'll be transforming him before he notices. You can't force someone to take an interest in himself and the world, but you can make it appealing and easy for someone who's too tired, too fed up, too dispirited and tuned out to do it for himself.

Changing a man's wardrobe is a lot easier than changing his attitude. Many men are naturally elegant dressers, having a

Menstyle

wonderful eye for suit fabric, the right shirts and all the trimmings. Some men begin adulthood as fashion plates and never give it up, looking at fifty, even sixty and beyond, absolutely great and *de rigueur* in an oversized Armani coat, N. Peal's cashmere polo-necks and suits from Ferre. Or maybe not. Maybe they turn the splashier elegance of their youth to a more traditional line, with Turnbull and Asser shirts and ties from Gieves and Hawkes. Or stay with their comfortable country elegance in corduroys, heavy sweaters and waxed jackets. The ease and comfort with which they wear their clothes makes for elegance as much as the fabric and style. Men's clothing has not changed as dramatically as women's in this century. Edwardian jackets and trousers still look recognisable and wearable where women's dresses of that period look like costumes. A man can look the picture of elegance in an out-at-the-elbows tweed jacket he's worn for thirty years and corduroy trousers almost as ancient. But the plastic mac, dark skinny tie and too short suit trousers have to go. All the outward dressing won't stand up as elegant if it isn't bolstered by an inner elegance as well. Men come into their own in the charm department as they get older, making them entertaining and treasured companions and lovers. With as much going for them as for women at this age, it's a wonder they ever agonise about lost youth and make misguided attempts to pursue it at all.

For both men and women, mid-life earns its reputation as a time of "crisis". Many couples find they can't weather the differences, not just because of what they've both become, but because of what they want to become and make with the rest, and best part, of their lives. Some women are taken by surprise when *he* leaves. Others feel their only route to fulfilment is to leave themselves, and remake a life, perhaps with another, different man.

It takes women a long time to understand men and decide what they want from them. Although interests change and personalities grow as you get older, you usually fall for the same type of man throughout your romantic life: an intellectual, a flatterer, a practical outdoorsman, a dreamer, a romantic – the same types keep coming up in your date-book again and again. Most women would say they want a man sensitive enough to be protective, but independent enough to let them follow their own interests. They want him to be attentive, but not jealous, experimental but disinclined to stray, funny but not a fool, open-minded but reliable, romantic and inclined to cherish what he's got. A man's list of what he wants in a woman would be just as long, but that's another story.

If women listed the top ten things about men that drive them mad and out the door, they'd be:

◆ Unreliability (he never calls)
◆ Absenteeism (every night at the pub, every Sunday on the pitch)
◆ Lying *("Honestly, it's a business trip")*
◆ Irresponsibility *("How did I know they weren't supposed to watch late movies on a school night?")*
◆ Helplessness (can't turn on the cooker or iron a shirt)
◆ Stuffiness (hates all music/movies/fashions/novels that have come out since he turned thirty-five)
◆ Dullness *("Sod those samosas or whatever you call them, give me a proper bit of meat and veg")*
◆ Laziness *("I don't care what you've read in those women's magazines, we've done it this way every Saturday night for twenty-five years")*
◆ Cruelty *("You look bloody ridiculous in those clothes")*
◆ Deafness (It is possible to pour your heart out to a man for an hour and he won't have taken in a single word).

This list of inelegant things makes it puzzling that women want anything to do with men, but that's because there's another list, the upside of a relationship in which all the tenderness, warmth, excitement, stimulation, comfort, support, fulfilment and satisfaction of being with a man rate highly.

Many women, whether they've become disillusioned with the man they've got or are looking for a replacement, torpedo any relationship with unrealistic expectations. To survive with your man of the moment, or any man of the future, an elegant woman has to extend understanding and generosity and a sense of fair play to him as much as she does to herself and her women friends.

◆ Show him you respect him and his work, whatever it is. Respect is very important to most men, and women who belittle their partners don't keep them for very long. Save the sarcasm for someone tougher than a man, someone who can take it – the cat maybe or a woman friend.

◆ It's unfair, unrealistic and inelegant to expect the man in your life to supply you with never-ending emotional and physical thrills and joy. He is not responsible for your happiness – you are – although he may be part of it. You both have exactly the same percentage of the relationship – so live up to your half.

◆ Resign yourself to the fact that your man has some fatal flaw – greediness, or stinginess, or a workaholic streak, or he eats peanut butter out of the jar. No one's perfect, but remember elegance isn't perfection either, it's ease with oneself and one's surroundings and tolerance of others' quirks and foibles.

◆ Honour his privacy. For a lot of women, being in love is twenty-four hours of "being there". That's not love, it's suffocation. Everybody, men and women, needs some breathing space and private time alone, away from the world, and that includes family and you. Don't begrudge him his afternoon walking or fishing, his evening hours with a hobby or book to himself. You don't have to share everything to share a life.

Women in good solid relationships with men have been doing this all along. It keeps a relationship strong and stable but fresh and satisfying at the same time. Respect for the individual within a twosome is very elegant.

But for women on their own, where will they look for and find an elegant man? Poaching someone else's is really not elegant. Elegant men come in all shapes and sizes, cross all social strata and have diverse interests, but are all full of the same elegant spirit that makes women so desirable and on their best form. Elegant men are strong enough for others to sense their inner strength, confidence and self-esteem and considerate enough to let others flex their own personality. An elegant man does not play the wounding, slighting games

beloved of insecure, weak and inelegant men. He does not, for example:
- ◆ Swear eternal love, then disappear for three weeks without so much as a phone call.
- ◆ Embarrass you in front of others with personal slights and asides.
- ◆ Speak for you, as in "Jane thinks that . . . Jane wouldn't agree with this . . ."
- ◆ Physically mistreat women.
- ◆ Collect women and broken hearts like butterflies, following a quantity not quality theory.
- ◆ Adore himself so much there's no attention left for anyone else.

Every woman knows or has known a man (or men – oh dear) like this. This is largely because women subscribe to the biggest myth in all dealings between the sexes, the myth that love will change someone, specifically that your love will change the one particular man you want. Weather changes, seasons change, fashion changes, but the inner man, never.

The object of love is not to remould the loved one, but to enjoy each other, faults included, offer kindness and comfort, support and respect and admiration. If a condition of love is that he must change, it isn't love – love doesn't have conditions, only tolerance and sensitivity to each other. Occasionally love may help someone change because he wants to change – perhaps you will help him fight a drinking problem, or give up smoking, or battle a workaholic drive – but the impulse has to come from him, not be part of your overall, remodelled, new improved design.

All your deepest, freely given love will not make an inconsiderate man thoughtful, a cruel man kind, or turn a puritan into a hedonist.

There are four other categories of men to avoid like the plague if you're looking for long-term love with an elegant man of your own.
- ◆ Violent men, no matter what excuses they offer of a miserable childhood, ungovernable temper, or their copious contrition afterwards, are not for any woman who values her physical and mental well-being, has a

Menstyle

strong sense of self-worth and puts a high value on herself.

◆ Gay men are always gay. Your love won't convert him, and no matter what good company he is, what a great cook, raconteur or how downright sexy he is, the match is off before it begins.

◆ Confirmed bachelors of a certain age like their single status and don't want a permanent partner disrupting their carved-in-stone routines, despite the way he seems to be wavering after a wonderful weekend away. You may get a visitor's pass but you'll never take up permanent residence.

◆ Married men, who want to remain married.

Finally, one of the keys to self-preservation is when a man tells you he's no good, believe him. It's the last honest thing you're likely to hear.

There are elegant unattached men out there but finding one can be tricky. Most women meet men at work or through friends, but increasingly single women have some success in more casual surroundings, such as walking the dog (easy and natural to greet a fellow stroller), wandering around galleries and museums, by joining clubs and groups – sailing and gardening seem especially worthwhile – and going to night classes, socially DIY and photography top the list.

Occasionally women who find themselves suddenly single get rid of a lot of the animosity, distrust and unhappiness of their previous relationship by working it out through a series of quick and casual affairs. As short-term therapy goes, it can be fun as long as you can still wink at yourself in the mirror in the morning and make sure you take precautions against the risk of AIDS. But sooner or later, most women will crave something more substantial, for what elegant women miss is not just the physical satisfaction but the warmth and affirmation of intimacy.

"*True,*" says a happily philandering woman, "*in the first year after my divorce, men were my favourite between-meal snack. But that kind of life wears thin. You're untouched emotionally and women need some emotional connection.*" Yes they do, and they need it from a loving and potentially long-term relationship. Women may be shy of starting over again, especially if they've been hurt by a previous relationship which ended badly, or shocked by premature widowhood. But if they're lucky enough to start again, they, and all women in established relationships, should do their elegant best to keep it going. Much of the life-force of long-term love comes from the elegant precepts of consideration, kindness and graciousness towards others, the confidence to express these feelings, and the self-esteem to expect and get them back in return. Love needs to be expressed verbally and physically. You can't tell someone you love them too many times. Physical affection doesn't mean passionate sex every night, but regular *touching* – brushing an arm in passing, a touch at the wrist, a brief hug when passing through the room – physical affirmation that you're there, you're together, with a great deal unspoken but not needing to be spoken, about the depth of feeling and need.

Mature women also know that relationships live longer when both of you concentrate on each other's strengths and goodness, not weaknesses and faults. The good things matter now, the failings can be swept away, they're no longer as important as you once thought they were. All couples need to consciously make time together. The busyness and speed of life swallow relationships whole. There are times when chores, work, family needs and the problems of the world need to be shoved aside and the two of you take precedence. Real love has a tough and realistic side. It can stand to know about all the things that go wrong, all the fears and insecurities, even the failures that won't diminish you in the eyes of someone who loves you. All elegant women know this. And all elegant men.

How to spot an elegant man across a crowded room
◆ He looks like he belongs
◆ He has a twinkle in his eye
◆ He's not checking his reflection in the mirror
◆ He's smiling at you

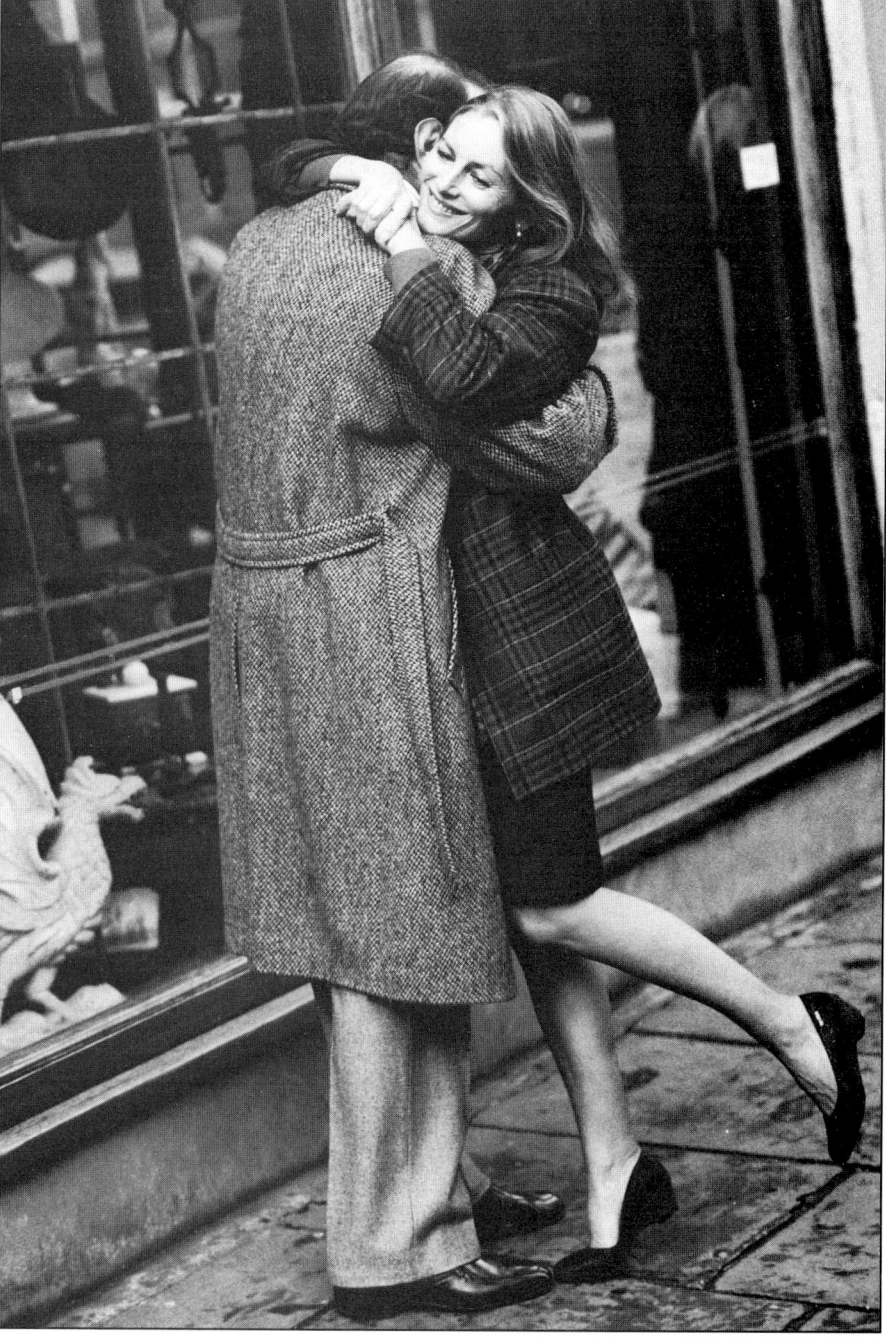

AN ELEGANT AFTERWORD

What use is all this elegance you've worked so hard to develop and achieve? Its obvious outward advantages are personal – the sense of well-being a woman has when she knows she looks wonderful, the acceptance and admiration good physical looks exact as their due. Inner qualities of elegance propel a woman with courage and dignity through the minefields of relationships and life's various triumphs and storms. In every situation she shines just that much brighter armed with confidence, self-assurance and ease, and a sense of her own capability. Her own elegance is a contribution to life's general pool of beauty and grace. When you're cultivating an elegant style, keep mind and spirit open to the elegance of life that surrounds you. There is much beauty, simplicity and complexity to feed the eye and soul in music, nature, landscapes and seascapes, art and architecture, and the kindness, talents and goodness of fellow travellers. The world is full of grandeur and grace, with much to imitate and much to uplift you. Feeling that so much good exists in a world relentlessly portrayed as gruesome and violent in the daily digest of news, is in itself beneficial. Behaviour is nurtured and inspired by many outside influences – your taste and elegance can find a hundred sources to turn to for inspiration, and from that inspiration you give something elegant back to yourself and to the world that inspired you.

AN ELEGANT AFTERWORD

No woman should ever feel her time of beauty – inner or outer – has passed. Women in the autumn of their lives, as this time is often described, captivated one of the most passionate and elegant poets in the English language: "No spring, nor summer beauty hath such grace, as I have seen in one autumnal face," *and nothing has changed in the several hundred years since John Donne expressed his devotion.*

There's something flattering and inspiring about autumn as a season. Spring is pale and untried, summer too obvious, winter too sparse, but autumn has just the right combination of strength and splendour, deep colour and mellowness too. Altogether a good season of life to celebrate.

Women put elegance to good use when they make their lives a reflection of "their" season: strong and splendid, colourful and rich, in every way. Elegance becomes a way of life, and is becoming to every woman.

THE ELEGANT QUIZ

A quick way to check your elegance quotient is by answering the following questions honestly with your *first*, unpremeditated response.

1   A beautiful woman wafts into the room at a large gathering; all heads turn. Do you immediately comment:
   a "What a lovely woman."
   b "Loved her dress *last* year too."
   c "Probably a man dressed up."

2   After passionate love-making with your man, do you mentally compare him to:
   a Harrison Ford
   b A Norwegian fjord
   c An old Ford Cortina

3   At a dinner party the chap seated next to you slips his hand on to your knee under the tablecloth. Do you:
   a Scream and upset the wine glasses
   b Stab him in the thigh with your salad fork
   c Sharply move your knee and tell him *sotto voce* that you're sure he was mistakenly reaching for his napkin, but if he so much as breathes in your direction again, you'll dump the *pappardelle al pâté di carciofo* all over his Armani-ed legs.

4   A friend has just got a stunning promotion at work. Do you:
   a Spread a rumour that all that sleeping with the boss finally paid off
   b Remind her that every management woman you've ever known has had her marriage end in divorce
   c Give a congratulatory lunch in her honour.

THE ELEGANT QUIZ

5 Do you admire the fashions of:
   a The early nineteenth century (the Regency)
   b The 1930s
   c The 1950s

6 You're squeezing into a party dress in the changing room of your favourite boutique but your bottom's bulging and you can't do up the zipper, not even before lunch and holding your breath. You decide:
   a You must go on a diet today
   b You must go on a diet tomorrow
   c You must get a larger size. Everyone gets bigger as they get older.

7 Your rich friend is giving a masquerade party for New Year's Eve. Are you going as:
   a Queen Elizabeth I
   b A queen bee
   c Queen Victoria

8 Your favourite suave and sensitive fictional detective is:
   a Hercule Poirot
   b Lord Peter Wimsey
   c Mike Hammer

9 Your daughter is going through a difficult time in her new marriage. Would you:
   a Say right out, she's made her bed and can lie in it
   b Tell her the whole family was against the marriage from the start and no one's surprised he's turned out a swine
   c Agree that all marriages go through rocky times and invite her to come and talk about it, or anything else, while she's sorting it out.

10 You're planning a get-together for four couples, all old friends, when one of the women rings up and says she and her husband have separated and she'll be coming alone. Do you face this awkwardness by:
   a Immediately ringing around everyone you know to find a suitable man of any age to make up the numbers
   b Ask her not to come because it will look so obvious and painful she's on her own
   c Serve a buffet rather than a sit-down dinner, so her solo appearance isn't so noticeable and awkward.

THE ELEGANT QUIZ

11 You redecorate your sitting room and invite a friend in to view it. She says "glad you like it but it doesn't appeal to me and it's gone right out of fashion." Do you think:
 a She's right, it's awful, I'll change it all
 b She's right, I'll have to wait till it comes into fashion again before I can have anyone over
 c She's wrong, it's timeless and I love it.

12 Now you're so slim you can wear blue jeans with pride, do you stick them on with footwear consisting of:
 a Flat shoes
 b High heels
 c Sandals with striped socks

13 Every woman needs time alone to reflect and recover, a place of peace and solitude. If you need a little privacy, do you:
 a Retreat to "a room of your own", or corner of a room that the family respects as yours and leaves you undisturbed
 b Lock yourself in the loo
 c Go out and wander around – there is no privacy at home.

14 You treat yourself to a vivid and uncharacteristic dress. Your husband remarks he's never seen you in that colour before. Your daughter opines it would fit her better. You take one look at yourself in the mirror, and:
 a Sigh and give it to your daughter
 b Agree you've never worn this colour before and if he thinks it's too vivid you'll put on the familiar black-and-white check instead
 c Agree you've never worn this colour before but it looks sensational and it fits you just fine.

15 Your husband grumbles that your part-time job means you're not home every evening to put dinner on the table. Do you:
 a Apologise and give the job up even though you enjoyed it
 b Start an argument and say for years he was never home to eat dinner anyway
 c Explain calmly that your job is important to you, and that he too can learn to operate a microwave or make a salad.

16 Friends from out of town phone at the last moment and say they're passing by and will drop in for a quick visit. You've hardly any food in the house. Do you:
 a Invent an excuse to be out for the evening and ask for a little more notice next time

b Send out for a pizza even though the local takeaway stuff is like soggy cardboard – at least it won't be your fault it's badly cooked

c Rustle up some sandwiches, cheese and biscuits, grab a handful of flowers from the garden, and be informal and enjoy the company.

17 In bed you call your partner by another name. Do you:
   a Wish you were dead
   b Wish you were dead
   c Wish you were dead.

18 You're considering returning to work, but after fifteen years at home, fear you may be past it. Do you believe it when you're told:
   a You're too old to go back
   b You're too unskilled to go back
   c You're just what they're looking for and there are many retraining programmes available.

19 You never finished university, but now the children have left home are tempted to take it up again. Are you doing it:
   a Despite the fact your husband says you get stupider as you get older
   b Despite the fact your children want you available to babysit, not busy studying
   c Because you love the subject and welcome the challenge of learning more.

20 Your besotted girlfriend brings her new beau to meet you. While she's out of the room, he makes a very heavy pass at you. Do you:
   a Immediately screech, order him out of the house and explain to your friend what's happened
   b Ring your friend that evening, explain what happened and advise she ditch him
   c Ring your friend, offer a gentle warning, without mentioning the actual pass, which you know will go unheeded, and stand by with a box of hankies for the inevitable bust-up.

THE ELEGANT QUIZ

Quiz answers

1 **a**-5 **b**-2 **c**-1	8 **a**-2 **b**-5 **c**-0	15 **a**-1 **b**-2 **c**-5
2 **a**-3 **b**-2 **c**-1	9 **a**-1 **b**-2 **c**-5	16 **a**-0 **b**-1 **c**-5
3 **a**-1 **b**-3 **c**-5	10 **a**-2 **b**-0 **c**-5	17 **a**-0 **b**-0 **c**-0
4 **a**-1 **b**-2 **c**-5	11 **a**-1 **b**-2 **c**-5	18 **a**-2 **b**-2 **c**-5
5 **a**-4 **b**-4 **c**-2	12 **a**-5 **b**-1 **c**-3	19 **a**-5 **b**-5 **c**-5
6 **a**-5 **b**-4 **c**-2	13 **a**-5 **b**-3 **c**-1	20 **a**-1 **b**-3 **c**-5
7 **a**-5 **b**-2 **c**-1	14 **a**-3 **b**-2 **c**-5	

If you scored between 80 and 100, you're an elegant woman, inside and out; between 60 and 80, you're on your way up to elegance; 40 to 60, you have a lot of elegant instincts, don't give up; below 40 – throw out those white stilettos, chewing gum and lava lamps, practise a little compassion, have some faith in yourself, and start again at the beginning of this book.

USEFUL ADDRESSES

If you want to find out more about any area that interests or concerns you – beauty, health, education, employment or lifestyle – the following organisations may be able to help.

Advisory Centre for Education, Fitzwilliam House, 32 Trumpington Street, Cambridge, CB2 1QY

Amarant Trust (help with understanding menopause and HRT), 80 Lambeth Road, London, SE1 7PW

British Medical Association, BMA House, Tavistock Square, London, WC1H 9JP

British Association of Aesthetic Plastic Surgeons, 35 Lincoln's Inn Fields, London, WC2

British Association of Cosmetic Surgeons, 17 Harley Street, London, W1

British Chiropractic Association, Premier House, 10 Greycoat Lane, London, SW1P 1SB

British Holistic Medical Association, 179 Gloucester Place, London, NW1 6DX

Association of British Correspondence Colleges, 6 Francis Grove, London, SW19 4DT

British Naturopath and Osteopathic Association, 6 Netherhall Gardens, London, NW3 5RR

British Society of Iridology, 40 Stokewood Road, Bournemouth, BH3 7NE

Cancer Research Campaign (for information on sun damage to skin), 2 Carlton House Terrace, London, SW1T 5AE

College of Reflexology, 50 Sydney Dye Court, Sporle, King's Lynn, Norfolk, PE32 2EE

Department of Education and Science (DES), Elizabeth House, 39 York Road, London, SE1 7PH

USEFUL ADDRESSES

Department of Employment, St Vincent House, 30 Orange Street, London, W2

Equal Opportunities Commission, Overseas House, Quay Street, Manchester, M3 3HN

Medau Society (nationwide information service), 8B Robson House, East Street, Epsom, Surrey, KT17 1HH (03727 29056)

National Back Pain Association, 31/33 Park Road, Teddington, Middlesex, TW11 0AB

National Osteoporosis Society, P.O. Box 10, Radstock, Bath, BA3 3YB

Relate (Head Office), Herbert Gray College, Little Church Street, Rugby, Warwickshire, CV21 3AP

Open University, Walton Hall, Milton Keynes, MK7 6AA

Optical Information Council, 57a Old Woking Road, West Byfleet, Surrey

Pilates, Alan Herdman Studios, 17 Homer Row, London, W1 (071-723 9953)

Return (Women returners training consultancy), 33 Lausanne Road, London, N8 0H3

Society of Homeopaths, 2 Artizan Road, Northampton, NN1 4HU

Society of Teachers of Alexander Technique, 10 London House, 226 Fulham Road, London, SW10 9EL

Vegetarian Society, Parkdale, Dunham Road, Altrincham, Cheshire

Women in Enterprise (when starting own business), St Gabriel's House, 24 Laburnum Road, Wakefield, WF1 3QS